Administering Medications

A Competency-Based Program for Health Occupations

Third Edition

Phyllis Theiss Bayt, R.N., B.S., C.M.A.

GLENCOE
McGraw-Hill

New York, New York   Columbus, Ohio   Mission Hills, California   Peoria, Illinois

Reviewers and Contributors

Kathryn E. DeSilva, Pharm. D.
Clinical Pharmacy Specialist, Infectious Diseases
James A. Haley Veterans' Affairs Hospital
Tampa, Florida

Barbara M. Lee, RN, BSN, CMA
Former Director, Medical Division
Midstate College
Peoria, Illinois

Bayt, Phyllis Theiss
    Administering medications : a competency-based program for health
occupations / Phyllis Theiss Bayt.—3rd ed.
        p.   cm.
    Includes bibliographical references and index.
    ISBN 0-02-800886-3 (student text).—ISBN 0-02-800887-1
(instructor's guide)
        1. Drugs—Administration.   I. Title.
    [DNLM: 1. Drugs—administration & dosage—programmed instruction.
QV 18 B361a 1994]
RM147.B39   1994
615'.6—dc20
DNLM/DLC
for Library of Congress   93-16412
                                                            CIP

Imprint 1996

Send all inquiries to:
Glencoe/McGraw-Hill
936 Eastwind Drive
Westerville, OH 43081

ISBN 0-02-800886-3 (Student Text)
ISBN 0-02-800887-1 (Instructor's Guide)

Printed in the United States of America.

5 6 7 8 9 10 11 12   POH   02 01 00 99 98 97 96

Contents

PREFACE

The growing importance of long-term health care facilities such as nursing homes and convalescent centers has prompted an ever-increasing demand for persons trained in the administration of medications. To meet this demand, there is a need for a compact, self-contained program of instruction that can be studied in a variety of settings—either in school or on the job—and that provides in one place the necessary information for understanding drug actions and procedures of administration.

This text is designed to meet this need. It is written for a diverse group of students including:

- students of health occupations in high schools, vocational schools, and community colleges;
- nurses needing a refresher course to take on new job responsibilities;
- technicians, home care/day care workers, and medical clerks who need to be familiar with medications;
- persons in emergency medical technician training programs;
- trainees in specialized long-term and acute care facilities such as nursing homes, alcoholic centers, hospices, and adult day care centers;
- practitioners in hospital inservice programs; and
- students in state-approved programs for medication assistants.

We recognize that administering medications is a serious responsibility requiring a thorough understanding of the basic concepts of drug action. To grasp these concepts further requires a certain background in normal body functioning and the changes caused by disease. Through the use of simplified language, profuse illustrations, and structured learning experiences, we have attempted to provide the necessary background and to make complex concepts accessible to students at varying educational levels. It is understood that the study of this text is to be supervised by a licensed physician or registered nurse, who is expected to guide and evaluate performance on specific administration procedures.

It is our hope that this text will build the solid foundation of understanding that enables students to administer medications competently, safely, and with proper attention to the needs of their patients.

INTRODUCTION

This textbook has been prepared to meet the requirements of competency-based education. This philosophy of learning and teaching has spread throughout the health fields. The term "competency-based" means making sure that all of you, as students, reach a certain level of ability (competence) in specific skills that are laid out as the goals of teaching and learning.

The specific skills you will learn are those required in the performance of certain duties and responsibilities. This contrasts with traditional instructional methods in which students are taught whatever the teacher feels is important and grades are assigned on the basis of how much they have learned.

However, in competency-based education, the goal is to make every student an "A" student. This is an appropriate goal in the health fields, where anything less than "A"-quality work is unacceptable.

You will notice the difference between competency-based and traditional instruction when you take the written and performance tests at the end of each unit. Competency-based education demands that you learn **everything** you need for the performance of your job. Therefore, to pass a written test, you must answer almost all the questions correctly. If you make too many errors, you will need to take the test again after additional study. The same is true of performance tests, in which you demonstrate practical skills for the instructor. You must carry out medication procedures correctly, efficiently, and with proper respect for the patient. Only when your work is of a high quality can you pass the performance test.

The aim of this textbook, then, is to ensure that you learn everything you need to know for the responsibility of administering medications.

Organization of Learning Materials

The text is composed of 18 chapters, each one covering a major topic in the administration of medications. Chapters 1 through 5 cover basic background information and routine procedures that are important for anyone who is responsible for medications in a hospital or clinical setting.

Chapters 6 through 15 deal with specific body systems and the drugs that affect each system. In these chapters you will learn something about the structure and function of body parts, about major diseases, and about types of drugs. You will also receive detailed instructions on how to give medications.

Chapters 16 through 18 cover special topics—how to give drugs by injection, drugs for anesthesia, and the problems and special needs of the elderly.

Each chapter is made up of several elements, each having a different purpose. The elements are described in the list that follows. Read through this section carefully to understand how the learning materials are organized.

Competencies At the beginning of each chapter is a list of competencies. These are detailed statements of things you will need to know or be able to do after studying the chapter.
Purpose: To alert you to key skills and facts to which you should pay particular attention as you read and study.

Vocabulary This is a list of the medical terms and other key words necessary for your understanding of the chapter content. These terms should be memorized. Most of the words are also defined in the text. This list is merely a study aid and a reference in case of questions.
Purpose: To pull together medical vocabulary in one place so that is is easier for you to study.

Text Presentation This is the main part of the chapter. It is a complete presentation of the material you need to learn to prepare for the practice procedures and to pass the written mastery test. This part of the chapter includes written text, tables, art, and other study aids. The text gives background information to help you understand new ideas and procedures. The headings of the various sections of the chapter serve as a guide to what is important to learn.

Purpose: To present the material to be learned in a brief, clear form. To give the necessary medical background for understanding procedures and ideas related to administering medications.

Chapter Reviews The Chapter Reviews cover all the important things you need to remember from the chapter. They include

- Using Medical Terminology
- Acquiring Knowledge of Medications
- Applying Knowledge—On the Job
- Using Resources—On the Job

Purpose: To reinforce the learning of new ideas and procedures and provide practice in applying certain procedures and skills in clinical settings.

Answers to Chapter Reviews Answers are given following each Chapter Review. The wording of the answers often differs from that of the text presentation, so that if something was not clear to you in the text, it may become clear when you read it in the answers.

Purpose: To give immediate feedback so that you know how well you are understanding the chapter content and to help you spot areas in which you need extra study.

Practice Procedures The practice procedures are a chance to practice the steps involved in administering medications. Your practice is guided by procedures that detail the steps in each task. The procedures are to be practiced under the supervision of an instructor or a nurse in charge. They can be carried out either in a teaching laboratory or on the job. It is expected that the supervisor will show you how to do them and give you tips on doing them well.

Purpose: To practice administering medications, under supervision, until you demonstrate that you are competent to administer them on your own.

Mastery Test This is your opportunity to show what you know. Each is a written test covering the chapter content. The 18 mastery tests are printed in the Instructor's Guide.

Purpose: To help you and your instructor find any weak spots in your knowledge that need extra study, and to prepare you for any licensing test you may need to take in order to be permitted to administer medications.

Performance Test Ten of the chapters call for a performance test, which is to be developed by your instructor or supervisor. The performance test is very important. It lets your instructor see whether you have reached the level of competence necessary for administering medications on your own to real patients. In the performance test, you should be able to administer medications skillfully and correctly.

Purpose: To make sure that you can perform the required tasks in a way that will benefit the patients who depend on your knowledge and skill.

How to Use This Text

This textbook contains all the learning materials needed for you to learn at your own pace. By studying the competencies, reading the text, and completing the chapter review and practice procedures, you will learn all you need to know to pass the mastery and performance tests. But to get the most out of the textbook, you need to know how to use it properly. Study this section very carefully, and refer to it often as you proceed through the book. The following list outlines the steps you should follow for each chapter.

1. Look at the competencies. They spell out the topics you should look for during your readings of the chapter. You may use the list of competencies as a sort of pretest to help you discover what you already know and what you need to learn. If you find you know most of the material in the chapter already, you can skip to the chapter review and the practice procedures and then take the mastery and performance tests.

2. Read through the vocabulary list. It contains important words that will be used to explain new ideas and procedures in the chapter.

3. Read through the text presentation fairly quickly. Your aim on this first reading is to get an overview of the chapter content.

4. Now study the chapter. Reread the text slowly, trying to remember as much as you can. Pay particular attention to the tables and charts. Some of these will need to be memorized.

5. Complete the chapter review. These will help you check how well you studied the chapter. They also require you to put your knowledge to work in realistic situations. If you have trouble with the exercises, go back and reread the relevant sections of the chapter. If you are still confused, consult your instructor, or look up the material in a reference book in the library.

6. Arrange to do the practice procedures in the laboratory or on the job, under the supervision of an instructor or a nurse in charge. Check to see whether the laboratory has special times set aside for students who wish to practice. Read through the procedure and then carry out the steps according to instructions.

    Your "patient" may be a plastic doll, a friend, or a real patient (under supervision only). Practice as many times as you need in order to do the tasks smoothly and carefully. Practice patience and thoughtfulness, even if your patient is just a plastic doll. Make your practice session as much like the "real thing" as possible. That way you will feel prepared when you must administer medications on your own.

7. Tell your instructor when you are ready to take the written mastery test. Find out whether there are certain hours when you can take the test in the library or the laboratory. Sign up for one of those times and then keep your appointment. Your test should be graded within a short time. To pass the test, you must not miss more than a few questions. Check with your instructor or laboratory coordinator for the percentage correct you need for a passing grade.

    After taking the test, find the answers to questions you missed. Remember, the idea is for you to learn everything you need to know to perform your job. If you missed more than the permitted number of questions, you will be required to repeat the test. Study the chapter again. To solve specific problems, consult a reference book or your instructor. Then retake the test. Go to Step 8 only when you have passed the mastery test.

8. Take the performance test. Inform your instructor that you are ready to demonstrate your skills and be evaluated. Sign up for a testing time and keep your appointment. Discuss your performance with the instructor. The instructor will judge the quality of your work. You must perform each task at a high level of skill in order to pass the performance test. Check with your instructor for the performance standards by which you will be evaluated. When you have passed the performance test, you may proceed to the next chapter and begin again at Step 1.

Tips on Individualized Study

- **Set yourself goals for study.**
  Without a plan, studying can drag out and take much longer than necessary. Check with your instructor or laboratory coordinator to see if a specific plan is to be followed in your course. If you are studying on your own, decide how many chapters you would like to complete each week or month. Then follow your plan. You will feel more confident about studying if you make steady progress through the materials.

- **Study with a friend.**
  Test each other on the vocabulary, drug information, body systems, diseases, and procedures. Talking about new ideas and procedures together helps both of you remember the material.

- **Use resources in addition to the textbook.**
  No textbook can fill the needs of every individual. Occasionally there will be topics you do not fully understand after reading the text. You can find other learning aids in the library or ask the instructor for help. Ask about audiovisual materials that are widely available for students of nursing and the health occupations. These demonstrate nursing procedures and give helpful hints on administering medications.

- **Take the chapter reviews and practice procedures seriously.**
  Do not dash through them or skip parts that seem hard or uninteresting. They are designed to give you needed practice in tasks that you will be performing on the job. They will also prepare you for the tests. The more you can rehearse the needed skills, the higher you will score on the tests and the more confident you will feel when you first take on your new responsibilities.

**C
H
A
P
T
E
R**

1

Orientation to Medications

◆◆ In this chapter you will learn where drugs come from, how they are standardized, and how their use is governed by law. You will also learn how to use drug references and drug cards to gather information about medications.

COMPETENCIES

After studying this chapter, you should be able to

- define pharmacology, pharmacodynamics, pharmacy, anatomy, physiology, and pathology.
- list the major sources of drugs and give examples of each.
- list the six therapeutic uses of drugs.
- define drug standards and tell how they are determined.
- explain why drug standards are necessary.
- list and describe four types of names by which drugs are known.
- name three drug references and show how to use at least one.
- use drug references to prepare a drug card.
- name three major drug laws and list their main features.
- name the federal agencies that enforce the drug laws.
- tell why health workers must be familiar with drug laws.

action: how a drug works

administration: how the drug is given

anatomy: the structure of body parts

chemical name: describes the chemical structure of a compound

contraception: the prevention of pregnancy

contraindications: conditions in which the use of a certain drug is dangerous or ill-advised

controlled substances: potentially dangerous or habit-forming drugs whose sale and use are strictly regulated by law

description: what the drug is made of

diagnostic drugs: help physicians determine if disease is present

drug: a chemical that affects the body

drug card: index card on which you write drug information for your own reference

Drug Enforcement Agency (DEA): enforces the Controlled Substances Act of 1970

FDCA: Food, Drug, and Cosmetic Act of 1938

Food and Drug Administration: enforcement agency for the FDCA

generic: any drug not sold under a particular product name

generic name: name provided for a new drug by the United States Adopted Names Council; a drug may have several product names but only one generic name

health maintenance: developing a healthy lifestyle; keeping existing diseases under control, and getting regular checkups

indications: diseases and disorders for which a certain drug may be used

legend drugs: prescription drugs

medication: drugs used for medical therapy

metabolism: chemical processes that take place in a human cell

narcotics: drugs that act on the central nervous system to produce euphoria (a false sense of well-being), drowsiness, and stupor; their use is subject to governmental control because they are dangerous and can cause chemical dependence or addiction

official name: drug name listed by the FDA and printed in the *United States Pharmacopeia/National Formulary (USP/NF)*

over-the-counter (OTC) drugs: drugs available without a prescription

package insert: printed information about the pharmaceutical product

pathology: changes in the body caused by disease

pharmaceuticals: drugs

pharmacodynamics: study of how drugs interact with body tissues

pharmacology: study of drugs (uses, preparation, routes, laws, etc.)

pharmacy: preparing and dispensing drugs; the place where a pharmacist works

Physicians' Desk Reference (PDR): a popular reference book that gives information about the drug products of major pharmaceutical companies

physiology: functioning of the body parts

precautions: warnings to use care when giving drugs under certain conditions

prescription drugs: a physician's written or verbal order that enables a person to purchase a drug from the pharmacy

product name: licensed drug name under which a drug prepared by a specific manufacturer is sold; also called brand, trade, or proprietary name

psychology: study of the mind

side effects: drug effects other than the desired beneficial ones

standards: rules ensuring uniform quality and purity

synthesized: drugs created in the laboratory from various chemicals

therapeutic drugs: drugs used to prevent, diagnose, and treat disease and to prevent pregnancy

therapy: treatment of disease or disorder

United States Adopted Names (USAN): organization that adopts the generic name of a drug

USP Drug Information for the Health Care Professional: Official reference for pharmacists or persons administering medications

USP/NF: *United States Pharmacopeia/National Formulary;* official book listing standardized drugs

INTRODUCTION

Not long ago, only doctors and nurses were allowed to administer medications. But times are changing; many others in the health occupations are now also asked to give or know about medications. They also are expected to observe how patients react after taking their medications. These are important new responsibilities. They demand that you, a member on the allied health team working with medications, also have knowledge of many health-related topics. You must know the basic principles of **pharmacology,** which is the study of drugs and their uses. You must understand how drugs interact with the human body, or **pharmacodynamics.** This requires some knowledge of human **anatomy,** the structure of body parts, and of **physiology,** the functions of body systems, organs, tissues, and cells. You must know what goes wrong with body parts when there is disease, or **pathology,** and how drugs change the course of disease. Attention must be given to **psychology,** the study of the mind, because the mental state of a patient influences the way the body reacts to drugs.

The units of this textbook will teach you, step by step, the basics of pharmacology, pharmacodynamics, anatomy, physiology, and pathology. Tips on how to respond to patients' psychological needs will be included. The uses of specific drugs for treatment of disease are discussed in connection with the parts of the body on which they act. As you learn general principles, a number of you will also carry out practice tasks to give you experience in giving medications.

PHARMACOLOGY

A **drug** is any chemical that affects living things. Pharmacology is the study of drugs: their sources, chemical makeup, preparation, and uses. Pharmacology includes the study of how specific chemicals affect the human body. In the field of medicine, we are concerned with drugs that help prevent, diagnose, and treat human disease. These are called **therapeutic drugs,** or **medications.**

Pharmacology attempts to describe both the desired effects and the side effects of drugs. It also focuses on the proper amounts of drugs to be given and on how drugs are given. Knowledge of the laws and responsibilities surrounding drug use, along with practical experience in giving medications, will equip you to play a vital role in the health care team.

DRUG SOURCES

Drugs come from four sources: plants, animals, minerals, and chemical synthesis/biogenetic engineering in the laboratory.

Our ancestors long ago discovered that the roots, leaves, and seeds of certain plants had the power to cure illnesses, ease pain, and affect the mind. Today many drugs are still extracted from parts of plants. An example is digitalis, which is used to treat certain heart conditions. Digitalis is made from a wildflower, purple foxglove. Other drugs and useful substances include opium, belladonna, vitamin C, and various gums and oils.

Drugs of animal origin are prepared by extracting natural substances, such as hormones, from animal tissues and organs. Insulin, for example, is extracted from the pancreas of cattle and pigs. Heparin, used to reduce the formation of blood clots, is taken from the intestinal linings of cattle and pigs.

Iron, iodine, calcium, and sodium chloride (salt) are examples of minerals used in drug therapy. They come from rocks and crystals found in nature.

Many drugs are made, or synthesized, in the laboratory through chemical processes. An example is hydrochlorothiazide *(HydroDIURIL)*, a drug used to treat high blood pressure. Biogenetic engineering methods, patching together DNA material from different organisms, have made new drugs and drug products available. Insulin and vaccines can be produced this way. Biogenetic engineering also involves taking a normal human substance and mass-producing it in animals, yeasts, and so on.

DRUG USES

The study of drug uses will give you an understanding of one phase of health care, drug therapy. Drugs are helpful to both the healthy and the sick. The four most familiar uses of drugs relate to disease: prevention, treatment, diagnosis, and cure. The last two uses of drugs are **contraception,** or the prevention of pregnancy, and **health maintenance.**

Disease prevention involves the administration of drugs such as vaccines that inoculate the body against disease germs. Health maintenance is closely related to disease prevention. Drugs such as vitamins and insulin are given to help keep the body healthy and strong or to keep the body systems functioning normally.

Treating disease means relieving the symptoms while the body's natural disease-fighting mechanisms do their work. Aspirin and antihistamines are examples of drugs used to treat disease symptoms. Curing disease often means eliminating disease-causing germs. Antibiotics such as streptomycin and penicillin are drugs that help cure disease.

Diagnostic drugs are taken to enable physicians to determine whether disease is present. For example, radiopaque dye (a dye that shows up on fluoroscopes or x-rays) is administered to detect gallbladder malfunctions.

The prevention of pregnancy is possible with the use of contraceptives, drugs that control fertility.

Drugs often have more than one use. The drug promethazine hydrochloride *(Phenergan)*, for example, is used in a wide variety of ways. It can control allergic reactions, treat motion sickness, induce sleep, and prevent vomiting after surgery. Some drugs have the ability to prevent as well as cure or treat disease. The uses of different kinds of drugs are discussed in specific units.

DRUG STANDARDS

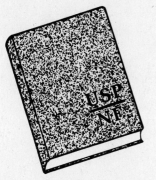

Figure 1-1 United States Pharmacopeia/National Formulary.

Drugs differ widely in strength, quality, and purity, depending on how they are manufactured. In order to control these differences, certain rules or **standards** have been set up that products must meet. Drug standards are required by law. The law says that all preparations called by the same drug name must be of a uniform strength, quality, and purity. A drug prepared in Indiana must meet the same standards for strength, quality, and purity as the same drug prepared in California or New Jersey. Because of drug standards, physicians who order penicillin, for example, can be sure that patients anywhere in the country will get the same basic substance from the pharmacist. Drug standards also help doctors prescribe accurate dosages and predict the results.

Drugs for which standards have been developed are listed in a special reference book called the **United States Pharmacopeia/National Formulary** (USP/NF) (Figure 1-1). The USP/NF is recognized by the U.S. government as the official list of drug standards, which are enforceable by the U.S. Food and Drug Administration.

Since 1975, USP has engaged in a program to include all drug substances and, to the extent possible, all drug products in the United States. The book is updated regularly, and a new edition is published every five years to keep the information up to date.

DRUG NAMES

All drugs have more than one name. In fact, most have four: a chemical name, a generic name, an official name, and one or more product names. Figures 1-2 through 1-5 on pages 6 and 7 show the four names of one common drug.

The **chemical name** describes the chemical structure of the drug. It can be very long and complicated.

The **generic name** is the name given a drug by the manufacturer with input from various regulatory agencies before the drug becomes officially recognized. It gives some information about the chemical makeup of the drug, but not as much as the chemical name. The generic name is established by the **United States Adopted Names (USAN) Council**. (The term **generic** has also come to mean any drug that is not sold under a particular product name.)

The **official name** is the name under which the drug is listed in the USP/NF. It is usually, but not always, the same as the generic name. If the USP/NF does change a name of one of its drugs, that name becomes the one and only allowable generic name in the United States.

Also known as the brand, trade, or proprietary name, the **product name** is the name under which the drug is sold by a specific manufacturer. The name is owned by the drug company, and no other company may use it. The symbol ® to the right of the name shows that its use is restricted. A drug that is manufactured by several companies may be known by several different product names. For example, the drug with the generic name nitroglycerin is sold by several manufacturers under such product names as *Nitro-Bid, Nitrong,* and *Nitrostat.*

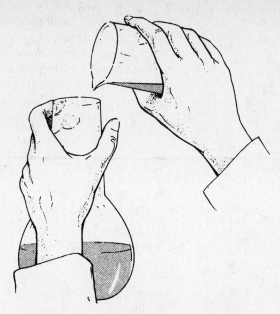

6-Chloro-3,4-dihydro-2H-1,2,4-
benzothiadiazine-7-sulfonamide
1,1-dioxide

Figure 1-2   Chemical name.

Product Name Drugs versus Generics

Most drugs are known to the general public by their product names. *Librium,* for example, is much more familiar to most people than chlordiazepoxide hydrochloride. But you and your fellow health workers must be familiar with the generic names of many drugs. There are good reasons for this. First, drugs are frequently prescribed by their generic names rather than by their product names. This is because the product name preparations are more expensive, so the consumer saves by buying generic drugs. In fact, state and federal governments now permit, encourage, and, in some cases, mandate that the consumer be given the generic form when buying prescription drugs. A prescription written for a generic product allows the pharmacist to choose among nonbranded drugs available from several companies. Bioavailability testing has helped to ensure that the patient gets the same benefits from the generic product as from the brand name product.

Another reason for knowing the generic name is that drugs often have several product names but only one generic name. (Did you remember the USP/NF allows only one in the United States?) If you learn the generic names, you can organize information about several product name drugs in your mind. Of course, it is not possible for you to memorize all of the generic and product names for medications, but you should try to become familiar with both names of the drugs you handle daily in your work.

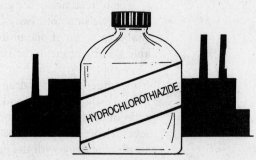

Figure 1-3   Generic name.

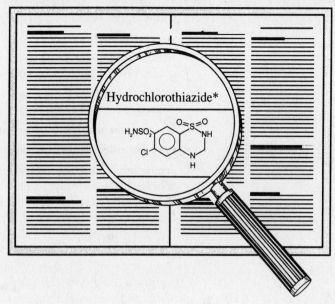

Figure 1-4 Official name.

Where specific drugs are mentioned in this text, generic names are given first and are not capitalized. Product names are capitalized and shown in parentheses in italic type following the generic names. Only one or two common product names are given in each case. Keep in mind that many other product name products may be available.

DRUG REFERENCES

Several reference books provide useful information about drugs on the market. These are often referred to by doctors, nurses, and others in the health occupations when planning and administering drug therapy. Drug references can help you understand why and how a particular drug is administered. For each drug, they usually include information about the following:

- **description**—what the drug is made of
- **action**—how the drug works

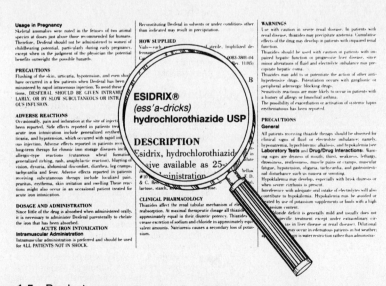

Figure 1-5 Product name. © Physicians' Desk Reference,® 1993, 47th Edition, published by Medical Economics Data, Montvale, New Jersey 07645. Reprinted by permission. All rights reserved.

- **indications**—what conditions the drug is used for
- **contraindications**—conditions under which the drug should not be used
- **precautions**—special conditions that may alter the drug's effects and that should be considered when prescribing the drug
- **adverse reactions**—unpleasant or dangerous effects of a drug other than the desired effect (see Chapter 2)
- **dosage and administration**—how the drug is given
- **how supplied**—how the drug is packaged and stored

Learning how to use the drug references will help you meet the new responsibilities of health workers in administering medications.

A popular reference book is **Physicians' Desk Reference** (PDR), which is available in most health facilities (Figure 1-6). The PDR gives information about the drug products of major pharmaceutical companies. It is useful for checking clinical pharmacology, mechanism of action, indications, contraindications, warnings, precautions, adverse reactions, overdosage, dosage and administration, and how the product is supplied. It lists drugs by their product, generic, and chemical names and manufacturers. Color photographs are included in a "Product Identification" section to help you identify some common drugs.

A new drug reference is the **USP, Drug Information for the Health Care Professional** (Volumes 1A and 1B, Volume II, and Volume III). The USP DI is written in everyday language. It provides pharmacists and other health care workers with easy-to-follow information on official drugs and products. You will find Volume II useful, as this volume is written especially for the patient. It is called *Advice for the Patient.* Volume III is the "Orange Book," *Approved Drug Products and Legal Requirements.* This volume includes state and federal requirements for prescribing and dispensing drugs. These volumes are updated each month in the *USP DI Update.*

Another valuable reference is the *Handbook of Nonprescription Drugs,* published by the American Pharmaceutical Association. Pharmacology textbooks and articles in nursing journals are also helpful sources of information. Some health care facilities keep their own reference lists of the drugs they use most often.

Recently, health care professionals have begun using the *American Hospital Formulary Service (AHFS) Information Book.* This book is updated yearly, and information is easily located with just one index in the rear of the book.

TERAZOL® 7
Vaginal Cream 0.4%
(terconazole)

INDICATIONS AND USAGE
TERAZOL 7 Vaginal Cream is indicated for the local treatment of vulvovaginal candidiasis (moniliasis). As TERAZOL 7 Vaginal Cream is effective only for vulvovaginitis caused by the genus *Candida,* the diagnosis should be confirmed by KOH smears and/or cultures.

ADVERSE REACTIONS
During controlled clinical studies conducted in the United States, 521 patients with vulvovaginal candidiasis were treated with terconazole 0.4% vaginal cream. Based on comparative analyses with placebo, the adverse experiences considered most likely related to terconazole 0.4% vaginal cream were headaches (26% *vs* 17% with placebo) and body pain (2.1% *vs* 0% with placebo). Vulvovaginal burning (5.2%), itching (2.3%) or irritation (3.1%) occurred less frequently with terconazole 0.4% vaginal cream than with the vehicle placebo. Fever (1.7% *vs* 0.5% with placebo) and chills (0.4% *vs* 0.0% with placebo) have also been reported. The therapy-related dropout rate was 1.9%. The adverse drug experience on terconazole most frequently causing discontinuation was vulvovaginal itching (0.6%), which was lower than the incidence for placebo (0.9%).

DOSAGE AND ADMINISTRATION
One full applicator (5 g) of TERAZOL 7 Vaginal Cream (20 mg terconazole) is administered intravaginally once daily at bedtime for seven consecutive days. Before prescribing another course of therapy, the diagnosis should be reconfirmed by smears and/or cultures and other pathogens commonly associated with vulvovaginitis ruled out. The therapeutic effect of TERAZOL 7 Vaginal Cream is not affected by menstruation.

Figure 1-6 Information from the PDR. © Physicians' Desk Reference® 1993, 47th Edition, published by Medical Economics Data, Montvale, New Jersey 07645. Reprinted by permission. All rights reserved.

Coping with Technical Language

A problem with many drug references is that they are written in complex language. They use medical terms that may be unfamiliar, especially to new students. The descriptions of drugs assume that the reader has a background in anatomy, physiology, diseases, and pharmacology.

An important aim of this book is to help you learn enough so that you can understand what you find in drug references. You will learn important technical terms, basic principles to help you understand how drugs work, and enough about various diseases so that the reason for giving a particular drug will become clear.

In the chapter Review there is an exercise in using the PDR. It could be used for any drug reference your agency has on hand. This may be the first time you have looked at a drug reference. Do not be worried if the words and descriptions seem completely unfamiliar. By the end of this course, you will probably be surprised at how much more material makes sense to you.

Coping with Changing Information

Information about drugs is constantly changing. New drugs appear all the time, and old drugs are taken off the market. Drug research turns up better ways of using drugs and administering them. This means that drug references can become outdated very quickly. Some reference publishers send out regular supplements with information updates. These should be checked along with the drug reference. Another place to look for current information on drug administration is the **package inserts.** These are printed sheets of information found inside the boxes in which drugs are packaged. This is the same information provided in the PDR.

This text will help you cope with changing information on drugs. After studying the various chapters, you will know general principles about groups or classifications of drugs. Any new information that becomes available should then fit easily into your general understanding of drugs.

PREPARING YOUR OWN DRUG CARDS

Because there are so many drugs and so much information about them, no one can expect to keep all of the important facts constantly in mind. Many health workers find it useful to prepare 5×7 inch index cards containing information about the drugs that they most often use in their work. This saves time, because they can find the information quicker in their card files than in a huge drug reference. Of course, the information on the cards must be updated regularly to remain current. **Drug cards** can be designed according to your own needs. However, they should include at least these entries (discussed more fully in Chapters 2 and 3):

- Drug name, both generic and product.

- Drug classification, or the group a drug belongs to, such as analgesics (pain relievers), antipyretics (fever reducers), antacids, laxatives, and so on (you will learn the basic drug classifications in later chapters).

- Forms in which the drug is available (tablets, capsules, etc.).

- Action, or how the drug interacts with the organs or systems that it is supposed to affect.

- Uses of the drug.

- Side effects and adverse reactions.

- Signs of drug poisoning (toxicity).

- Route of administration.

- Dosage range and usual adult dose.

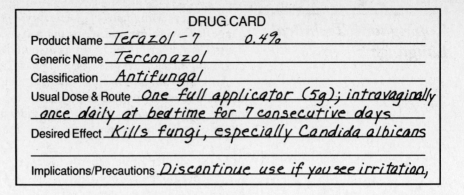

DRUG CARD

Product Name _Terazol - 7   0.4%_

Generic Name _Terconazol_

Classification _Antifungal_

Usual Dose & Route _One full applicator (5g); intravaginally once daily at bedtime for 7 consecutive days_

Desired Effect _Kills fungi, especially Candida albicans_

Implications/Precautions _Discontinue use if you see irritation,_

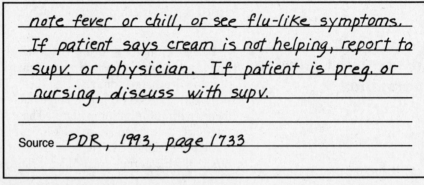

note fever or chill, or see flu-like symptoms. If patient says cream is not helping, report to supv. or physician. If patient is preg. or nursing, discuss with supv.

Source _PDR, 1993, page 1733_

Figure 1-7 Front and back of sample drug card.

- Special instructions for giving the medication, including nursing care required, what to tell the patient about expected side effects and precautions, and so on.

- A note on where you got your information (specific drug reference, package insert, etc.).

A sample drug card is shown in Figure 1-7. Beginning in Chapter 6, you will find product information tables listing representative drugs in the major drug categories. These tables can serve as a guide for what to include on your drug cards. As you study the drugs in Chapters 6 through 18, make a habit of preparing drug cards for the medications you expect to be giving in your own health facility.

DRUG LEGISLATION

The U.S. government regulates the composition, uses, names, labeling, and testing of drugs. Since the early 1900s, many laws have been passed to enforce the official drug standards and to protect the public from unreliable and unsafe drugs. Federal agencies have been set up to see that these laws are followed. Table 1-1 lists the major drug laws and their enforcing agencies.

The first law, the **Pure Food and Drug Act,** was passed in 1906. This law states that only drugs listed in the USP/NF may be prescribed and sold because these meet the required standards. Various amendments to this act regulate prescriptions, require the testing of new drugs, and call for complete information on drug effects and dangers. **The Food, Drug, and Cosmetic Act** (FDCA) of 1938, which replaced the 1906 act, spells out added regulations concerning the purity, strength, effectiveness, safety, labeling, and packaging of drugs. It also states that the government must review safety studies on new drugs before they can be put on the market. This provision was added after more than 100 deaths resulted from a poorly tested and mislabeled sulfanilamide product. The FDCA is enforced by the **Food and Drug Administration** (FDA).

Since 1962, the FDA has required proof that new drugs are effective as well as safe.

Another important law is the **Comprehensive Drug Abuse Prevention and Control Act of 1970.** It identifies the drugs that are dangerous or subject to abuse, such as narcotics, depressants, stimulants, and psychedelic drugs. The law states that the manufacture, distribution, and dispensing of these drugs must be controlled.

TABLE 1-1 Major Drug Laws

LEGISLATIVE ACT	ENFORCEMENT AGENCY
Pure Food and Drug Act of 1906 Approves USP/NF and requires that drugs meet official standards Requires labeling of medicines containing morphine Amendment of 1912 prohibits making false claims about health benefits of a drug	None
Food, Drug, and Cosmetic Act (FDCA) of 1938 (replaced the 1906 act) Regulates content and sales of drugs and cosmetics Requires accurate labeling and warnings against unsafe use Requires government review of safety studies before selling new drugs Amendment of 1952 allows certain drugs to be dispensed by prescription only, and to be refilled only on a doctor's order; also recognizes OTC drugs as drugs that do not require a prescription Amendment of 1962 requires proof of effectiveness and safety before marketing new drugs and full information on advantages, side effects, and contraindications Certain drugs must carry the label "Caution: Federal law prohibits dispensing without a prescription"	**Food and Drug Administration (FDA)** Under the Department of Health and Human Services Can investigate manufacturers, withdraw approval of drugs, and control shipment and testing Enforces FDCA by prosecuting offending firms and seizing goods Drug manufacturers must register with the FDA and report to the FDA all adverse reactions resulting from the use of their products Reviews studies of the safety and effectiveness of new drugs
Controlled Substances Act of 1970 Identifies and regulates manufacture and sale of narcotics and dangerous drugs Provides funding for education on drug abuse, rehabilitation of addicts, and law enforcement Classifies drugs into Schedules I–V according to medical usefulness and possible abuse (see Table 1-2)	**Drug Enforcement Administration (DEA)** Under the Department of Justice May punish violators by fines, imprisonment, or both
Drug Regulation and Reform Act of 1978 Permits briefer investigation of new drugs, allowing consumers access in a shorter time	FDA
Orphan Drug Act of 1983 Speeds up drugs' availability for patients with rare diseases	FDA
Drug Price Competition and Patent Term Restoration Act of 1984 Permits generic drug companies to prove bioequivalence without duplicating costly clinical trials done by the original drug manufacturer. Also gives longer patent protection for new drugs.	FDA

Otherwise, people might use these drugs carelessly and be injured physically or mentally.

Controlled substances are grouped into five categories or schedules, and each schedule has its own special restrictions, as shown in Table 1-2. A record is kept each time a controlled substance is sold, noting how much of the drug was sold. There are restrictions on how often and how prescriptions can be refilled. All prescriptions must be written in ink. Oral emergency orders for Schedule II substances may be filled, but the physician must provide a written prescription within 72 hours.

Pharmacists must follow carefully the rules outlined in the Controlled Substances Act. Violation of the law is punishable by fine or imprisonment or both. The agency that enforces this act is the **Drug Enforcement Administration** (DEA).

TABLE 1-2   Drug Classifications under the Controlled Substances Act of 1970[a]

Schedule I Drugs

High potential for abuse
To be used for research only
Not to be prescribed, as unsafe in treatment

Examples: alfentanil, fenethylline, hashish, heroin, lysergic acid diethylamide *(LSD)*, marijuana, **methaqualone** *(Quaalude)*, peyote, psilocyn

Schedule II Drugs

High potential for abuse; severe physical and psychological dependence
Acceptable medical uses, with restrictions
Dispensed by presciption only
No refills without a new written prescription from the physician

Examples: amphetamines, cocaine, meperidine HCl *(Demerol)*, methadone, methylphenidate hydrochloride *(Ritalin)*, morphine, opium, pentobarbital *(Nembutal)*, anabolic steroids

Schedule III Drugs

Moderate potential for abuse, psychological dependence, low physical dependence
Acceptable medical uses
By prescription only; may be refilled five times in 6 months if authorized by the physician

Examples: barbiturates, butabarbital *(Butisol)*, glutethimide *(Doriden)*, phendimetrazine *(Bacarate, Bontril PDM)*, secobarbital *(Seconal)*, *Tylenol* with codeine

Schedule IV Drugs

Lower potential for abuse than Schedule III drugs; limited psychological and physical dependence
Acceptable medical uses
By prescription only; may be refilled five times in 6 months if authorized by the physician

Examples: chloral hydrate *(Noctec)*, chlordiazepoxide *(Librium)*, diazepam *(Valium)*, flurazepam HCl *(Dalmane)*, oxazepam *(Serax)*, phenobarbital, propoxyphene HCl *(Darvon)*

Schedule V Drugs

Low potential for abuse
Acceptable medical uses
OTC narcotic drugs, but sold only by registered pharmacists; buyer must be 18 years and show ID

Examples: cough syrups with codeine, e.g, guaifenesin *(Naldecon DX)* and *Cheracol* with codeine, diphenoxylate HCl with atropine sulfate *(Lomotil[b])*, *Novahistine* expectorant, *Parepectolin*

---

[a]   Source: DEA, U.S. Department of Justice. Check with your local DEA office for current regulations.

[b]   Requires a prescription.

Doctors must also follow the law in prescribing controlled substances. They need a special license that is obtained from the DEA for each office from which they practice and must renew or register this license each year. They are given one tax stamp and number for each license. This number, called the DEA number, must be shown on any prescription for controlled substances.

In order to keep a supply of controlled substances in an office or a health facility, the staff must fill out special order forms and records. These forms show how many controlled substances are being kept at the facility, as well as who received doses of the drugs and how unused doses were disposed of. Every two years a physical inventory of all controlled substances in the office must be made. You will learn about these forms when you study Chapter 5.

◆ **NOTE** ◆ ◆ ◆ ◆ ◆ ◆ ◆ ◆ ◆ ◆ ◆ ◆ ◆ ◆ ◆ ◆

Be sure you understand these terms:

* **controlled substances**—drugs that have special restrictions on who can prescribe and sell them and on how often they can be prescribed.
* **OTC drugs**—can be bought and sold without a prescription.
* **prescription drugs**—must have a doctor's prescription (either oral or written) in order to be bought and sold; also called legend drugs.

YOU AND THE LAW

As a member of the health care team, you are responsible for knowing the laws controlling drug use and the regulatory agencies, i.e., the Federal Trade Commission (FTC) and the Consumer Product Safety Commission. The latter commission enforces the Poison Prevention Packaging Act (PPPA), which "child-proofs" drug packaging. Claiming ignorance of the law will not stand up in court if you are ever accused of irresponsible handling and administration of drugs.

How can you be sure you understand the law? As a first step, study carefully Tables 1-1 and 1-2. These summarize a great deal of information about the federal drug laws. You should be aware that the specific drugs under each schedule in the Controlled Substances Act may change. Your health facility will have an up-to-date list of controlled substances from the DEA. Get copies of federal drug laws from the library or from the FDA.

As a next step, you should study the laws of your state. These regulate such things as who may give medications, what kinds of training and supervision are required, who may keep the records, and who may take down prescriptions over the phone.

Your own health agency will also have regulations for you to follow. There will be special rules, for example, if your agency receives Medicaid or Medicare funds from the government. You should also find out the lines of authority in your agency—in other words, who is in charge of what and who supervises whom. That way, you can go to the right person when you have a legal question about giving a certain drug.

By knowing the law, you protect yourself from errors and possible lawsuits. But there is a more important benefit—the safety of your patient. By showing your awareness of drug laws, you help to educate your patients. You also gain their cooperation in following the laws. Drug laws are designed to protect the public. They depend on your example and your support.

Using Medical Terminology

Define each of the terms listed below.

1. Drug _____

    _____

2. Pharmacology _____

    _____

3. Pharmacodynamics _____

    _____

4. Anatomy _____

    _____

5. Physiology _____

    _____

6. Psychology _____

    _____

7. Drug standards _____

    _____

8. Drug references _____

    _____

9. PDR _____

    _____

10. *USP Drug Information for the Health Care Professional* _____

    _____

11. USP/NF _____

    _____

12. Pathology _____

    _____

13. Metabolism _____

    _____

14. USAN _____

    _____

15. Pharmacokinetics _____

    _____

    _____

    _____

Acquiring Knowledge of Medications

Answer the following questions in the spaces provided.

16. Name four sources of drugs, and give an example of a drug that comes from each source.

    Source   Example

    _____   _____

    _____   _____

    _____   _____

    _____   _____

17. Name the six therapeutic uses of drugs. Give examples.

    Use   Example

    _____   _____

    _____   _____

    _____   _____

    _____   _____

    _____   _____

    _____   _____

18. Why do you suppose we have drug standards and drug laws? Try to imagine what the medical field would be like without them.

    _____

    _____

    _____

    _____

    _____

    _____

19. Name the three major drug laws and the agencies that enforce them.

    Law and Date   Enforcing Agency

    _____   _____

    _____   _____

    _____   _____

    _____   _____

20. Differentiate between these legal classifications for drugs.

    OTC drugs _____

    _____

    prescription drugs _____

    _____

    controlled substances _____

    _____

From Column 2, select the term or phrase that best matches each item in Column 1.

Column 1

_____ 21. Chemical name

_____ 22. Generic name

_____ 23. Product name

_____ 24. Assay

_____ 25. Bioassay

_____ 26. Routes of administration

_____ 27. USP/NF

_____ 28. PDR

_____ 29. USAN

_____ 30. Official name

Column 2

a. *Visine* eyedrops

b. finding the therapeutic dose by testing a drug in animals, human volunteers, or isolated tissue

c. hydrochlorothiazide

d. methods of giving drugs

e. 6-chloro-3,4-dihydro-2H-1,2,4-benzothiadiazine-7-sulfonamide 1,1-dioxide

f. identifying and measuring ingredients in a laboratory

g. contains information about drug products provided by pharmaceutical companies

h. contains descriptions of official drugs and standards

i. name of drug listed in USP/NF

j. system that adopts generic names

Match the drugs to their schedules or classes as spelled out in the Controlled Substances Act of 1970.

Schedule

_____ 31. I

_____ 32. II

_____ 33. III

_____ 34. IV

_____ 35. V

Drugs

a. some barbiturates, *Doriden, Tylenol* with codeine

b. opium, morphine, *Demerol,* amphetamines, *Nembutal*

c. cough syrup with codeine, *Lomotil, Novahistine* expectorant

d. *Librium, Valium,* phenobarbital, *Noctec, Dalmane, Darvon*

e. heroin, hashish, LSD, peyote, alfentanil

Applying Knowledge on the Job

Respond to the following situation in the space provided.

36. Janie has just been hired for a new job in a nursing home. She wants to make sure that she knows what she is and is not allowed to do with regard to giving medications. What advice would you give her?

_____

_____

_____

_____

Using Resources on the Job

Obtain a current copy of the PDR and a medical dictionary from your school, nursing unit, or clinic. Use them to answer the questions that follow.

37. You are giving Mr. Jones regular-strength Tylenol every few hours after surgery. You would like to know something more about the drug, so you consult the PDR. Tylenol is a product name. Find the section in the PDR that lists drugs alphabetically by product names. What color are the pages?

_____

The PDR is divided into seven sections:
Manufacturer's Index (white pages): Names and addresses of drug companies, along with a list of drugs manufactured by each company.
Product Name Index (pink): Drugs listed alphabetically by generic/chemical and product names.
Product Category Index (blue): Drugs grouped according to their effects (e.g., analgesics, anesthetics, decongestants).
Generic and Chemical Name Index (yellow): Product names grouped under their generic or chemical names.
Product Identification Section (glossy): Full-color photograph and page numbers of selected medications, a quick reference for routine identification or in case of overdose or accidental poisoning.
Product Information (white): Main part of the book; gives detailed information about drug products, listed alphabetically by drug company.
Diagnostic Product Information (green): Special section for drugs used to diagnose diseases.

38. Look up Tylenol in the section you turned to in question 37. How many different forms of *Tylenol* are listed there? _____ Is there a small diamond to the left of any *Tylenol* form? If so, that means there is a photograph of it in the "Product Identification" section. Find the photograph.

39. Using the page number given for *Tylenol* tablets, look them up in the "Product Information" section. The generic name is listed just after the word *"Tylenol."* What is it?

_____

40. Read the description of Tylenol tablets. What kinds of information are given about the product?

_____

_____

_____

41. Under "Actions," *Tylenol* is described as an analgesic and an antipyretic. Look these words up in a medical dictionary and define them in your own words.

a. Analgesic _____

b. Antipyretic _____

42. Look at the section marked "Indications." List the conditions for which *Tylenol* might be ordered. (Use a medical dictionary if you need help to understand the technical terms.)

_____

_____

_____

43. Look at the section called "Precautions, Adverse Reactions or Warnings." What are the side effects of *Tylenol?*

_____

44. What is the usual adult dose of *Tylenol* tablets? _____

45. *Tylenol* tablets come in containers of various sizes. Find the section that tells you what sizes are available. List the sizes.

_____

_____

46. Look up the drug simethicone in the "Generic and Chemical Name Index." Under it you will find a list of products containing simethicone. Look up one of these products and find the following information:

Product headings _____

_____

Actions _____

_____

Indications _____

_____

Adverse reactions_____

_____

Dosage_____

_____

How supplied _____

47. Mrs. Allen has a skin condition called eczema. Her doctor has ordered *Cortisporin* ointment to help heal the dry, flaky sores (lesions) on her arms. Use the PDR to help you find out how to apply this ointment.

_____

_____

_____

48. *Tranxene* has been ordered for an elderly patient in the nursing home. What starting dosage is recommended in the PDR for an elderly patient for relief of anxiety?

_____

_____

_____

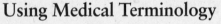

➤ **ANSWERS TO CHAPTER 1 REVIEW** ◀

Using Medical Terminology

1. Any chemical that affects living things, including the human body.

2. The study of drugs: sources, chemical makeup, uses, how to prepare them, and so on.

3. What happens when drugs interact with the cells of the human body.

4. The structure of the body and its parts.

5. How body systems, organs, tissues, and cells work.

6. The study of the mind, how people think, people's emotions, and so forth.

7. Rules concerning the strength, quality, and purity of drugs.

8. Books that give information about drugs.

9. *Physicians' Desk Reference,* a drug reference.

10. A drug reference for persons administering medications.

11. *United States Pharmacopeia/National Formulary,* a drug reference containing the standards for official drugs.

12. Study of the changes in the body caused by disease.

13. Chemical processes that take place in a cell.

14. *United States Adopted Names,* a system for adopting generic drug names.

15. The study of the drug movement into and out of the body.

Acquiring Knowledge of Medications

16. Drug sources include:
    - Plants—digitalis, opium, belladonna, vitamin C, gums, oils.
    - Animals—insulin, heparin.
    - Minerals—iron, iodine, salt, calcium.
    - Chemical synthesis—hydrochlorothiazide. *(HydroDiuril);* biogenetic engineering—insulin, vaccines.

17. Drug uses (may be answered in any order):
    - Prevent diseases—vaccines.
    - Maintain health—insulin, vitamins.
    - Diagnose disease—radiopaque dye, barium.
    - Treat disease—aspirin, antihistamines.
    - Cure disease—antibiotics.
    - Prevent pregnancy—contraceptives.

18. Answers will vary.

19. Drug laws and agencies:
    - Pure Food and Drug Act of 1906, no agency.
    - Food, Drug, and Cosmetic Act of 1938, enforced by the FDA.
    - Controlled Substances Act of 1970, enforced by the DEA.

20. OTC drugs can be bought and sold without a prescription. Prescription drugs need a doctor's written or verbal order to be bought and sold. Controlled substances have restrictions on who can prescribe, how, and how often.

21. e	22. c	23. a	24. f	25. b
26. d	27. h	28. g	29. j	30. i
31. e	32. b	33. a	34. d	35. c

Applying Knowledge on the Job

36. Janie should study the federal and state laws controlling medication administration. She should also study the nursing home's own regulations, and she should find out who is in charge so that she knows to whom questions should be addressed.

Using Resources on the Job

37. Pink

38. About 17 (this will vary from year to year).

39. Acetaminophen.

40. Description, actions, indications, precautions, adverse reactions, usual dosage, overdosage, how supplied.

41. a. Pain reliever.
    b. Fever reducer.

42. Pain of arthritis and rheumatism, headache, muscle pain (myalgia), nerve pain (neuralgia), menstrual cramps (dysmenorrhea), discomfort, and fever of colds.

43. Side effects are rare.

44. One or two tablets every 4–6 hours, no more than 12 per day.

45. Tins of 12; bottles of 24, 50, 100, and 200 tablets.

46. Answers depend on the product selected.

47. Apply a thin film to the affected area two or three times daily.

48. Dosage: 7.5–15 mg.

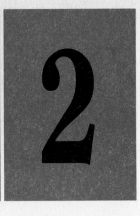

Pharmacodynamics

◆◆   In this chapter you will learn what happens to drugs when they enter the human body and how they produce their effects. You will study how drugs are affected by normal body processes, by characteristics of individual patients, and by the method and time of administration. You will also become familiar with the adverse reactions that can occur with drug administration.

COMPETENCIES

After studying this chapter, you should be able to

- state the four basic drug actions.
- name and describe the four body processes that affect drug action.
- identify at least 10 factors influencing drug action.
- differentiate between systemic and local drug effects.
- state the difference between the main effect and side effects.
- recognize descriptions of major adverse reactions.
- explain the difference between psychological and physical drug dependence.
- list the symptoms of withdrawal.
- state the health worker's responsibilities with regard to adverse reactions, drug dependence, and drug abuse.

absorption: passage of a substance into the bloodstream from the site of administration

action: the chemical changes in body cells and tissues caused by a drug

adverse reactions: dangerous or unexpected effects of drugs

allergy: reaction of the body cell to a foreign substance (antigen) to which it has previously developed antibodies; also called hypersensitivity

antagonism: two drugs acting together to cause a lesser response than the sum of their individual effects

antibody: a substance produced in the body that helps the body fight off foreign invaders like germs and antigens

antigen: substance that stimulates the production of antibodies and causes allergic reactions

biotransformation: normal body process by which substances are chemically broken down into a form that the body can excrete; part of the cells' work of burning fuel for growth and energy; also known as metabolism

capillaries: tiny blood vessels with very thin walls that let certain substances pass through them

cumulation: collection of drugs in the body due to slow biotransformation or slow excretion

dependence: a compulsion to continue taking a drug; can be physical and/or psychological

distribution: transport of drugs to body cells and spaces between cells

drug abuse: taking drugs for their mind-altering effects or taking too many drugs or too much of a drug

drug hypersensitivity: an allergic reaction to a drug that develops over time

drug misuse: overuse or careless use of any drug

dyspnea: difficult or labored breathing

edema: fluid collecting in body tissues

effect: a physical or psychological change in the patient brought about by a drug

enzyme: a chemical that speeds up biotransformation

excretion: the removal of waste substances from the body

habituation: drug dependence characterized by psychological dependence

histamine: substances released from injured cells during an allergic reaction, responsible for allergic symptoms

idiosyncrasy: a peculiar, unusual individual response to a drug

local: having an effect in the nearby area; for example, eyedrops designed to affect only the eye

main effect: the therapeutic effect for which a drug is administered

metabolism: also known as biotransformation

overdose: drug dose that is too large for a person's age, size, or physical condition

placebo effect: a therapeutic effect that results from a patient's belief in the benefits of a medication (a placebo can be a pill containing sugar or an injection of normal saline/sterile water)

potentiation: two drugs acting together to cause a greater response than the combined effects of each drug taken separately; also called synergism

reservoir: a tissue where drugs tend to collect; different drugs tend to collect in different tissues

side effects: drug effects that are not part of the treatment goal

systemic: having an effect throughout the body

tolerance: resistance to the effect of a drug

toxic: poisonous

withdrawal symptoms: set of physical reactions that occur when a person stops taking a drug on which he or she is physically dependent

PHARMACODYNAMICS AND BODY CELLS

Pharmacodynamics is the interaction between drugs and living things such as the human body. It refers to the chemical changes that drugs cause in the body cells and how those chemical changes alter body functions. The term *drug action* is used to describe the way drugs cause chemical changes in body cells. Drug effects are the physical changes that occur in the body as a result of the drug action.

To understand pharmacodynamics, you need to know something about cells. Cells are the basic building blocks of all living things, including the human body. Although cells work together in groups, each cell does certain routine things on its own to keep itself alive. Like all living things, it needs food and must eliminate waste materials. Human cells take in oxygen and nutrients, and they eliminate carbon dioxide and waste liquids.

Cells are very tiny; there are millions of them in the human body. If you look at a cell under a microscope, you can see the parts that carry out the routine jobs that keep the cell alive (Figure 2-1).

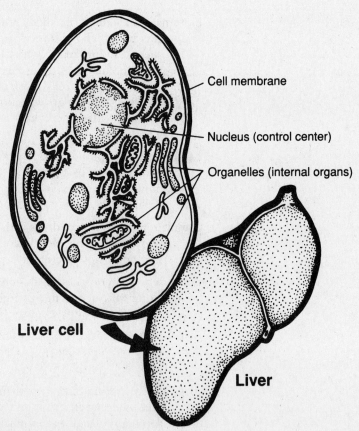

Figure 2-1 Diagram of a liver cell.

There are many different types of cells in the human body. Body organs and tissues are made up of similar cells held together by a special gluelike substance. These similar cells work together to carry out the jobs that organs and tissues must perform. For example, the liver is composed of specially designed cells that together perform the functions of the liver.

When a person takes a drug, the outcome depends on how that drug affects one or more groups of body cells. As you study pharmacodynamics, keep in mind that drugs always act on body cells in some manner.

DRUG ACTION

Drugs are chemicals that are known to have specific effects on the body. When one of these chemicals comes in contact with body cells, it causes changes in the cell molecules. That is, the chemical combines with or alters the molecules in body cells so as to change the way the cells work (Figure 2-2).

Drugs do not cause cells to function in entirely new and different ways, however. Usually they either slow down or speed up the ordinary processes that the cells carry out. For example, antihistamines slow the body's natural reactions to irritation, and stimulants speed up the energy-producing functions of cells.

Some drugs destroy certain cells or parts of cells. For example, some antibiotics kill disease germs, and fluorouracil and radioisotopes of cobalt kill cancer cells. Other drugs act to replace or supplement natural substances that the body

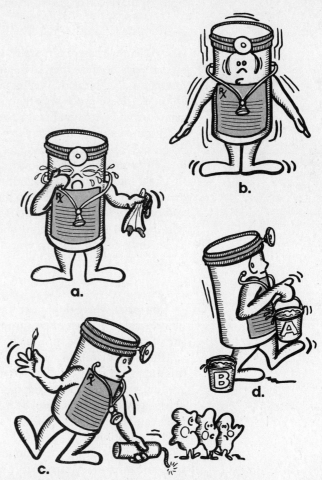

Figure 2-2 The four drug actions: a. depressing, b. stimulating, c. destroying cells, or d. replacing substances.

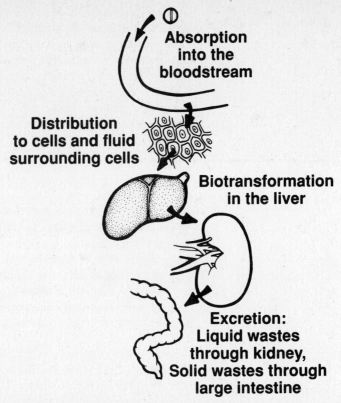

Absorption into the bloodstream

Distribution to cells and fluid surrounding cells

Biotransformation in the liver

Excretion: Liquid wastes through kidney, Solid wastes through large intestine

Figure 2-3   How a drug is handled by the human body.

lacks because of an organ malfunction or poor nutrition. Insulin is a drug taken by diabetics because they lack natural insulin.

Once a drug is taken, it enters into certain processes that go on in the body at all times. These processes are the body's normal means of using food and oxygen to produce energy. Energy is needed for cell growth and repair, for warmth, and for movement. Drugs are treated just like any other substance that enters the body, such as food, drink, and air. The only difference is that each drug interacts in a different way with the normal processes carried on by body cells.

These interactions are determined by many things: the size and shape of the drug molecules, their ability to dissolve in water or fat, the pH balance of drugs and cells, and the electrical charges of molecules. The details need not concern you, but you should have an understanding of four basic body processes that affect drug action: absorption, distribution, biotransformation, and excretion (Figure 2-3).

Absorption

No matter where they enter the body, sooner or later most drugs pass into the bloodstream and then move throughout the body. The passage of a drug from the site of administration into the bloodstream is called **absorption.**

Unless the drug is properly absorbed, it may not reach the organs or tissues that it is supposed to affect. The speed of absorption and the amount of absorption are important in pharmacodynamics. Drug action depends on how quickly and completely the drug is absorbed. When an exact serum level is important, blood tests can be ordered to find out how much drug is present in the bloodstream after absorption.

The type of drug, the amount of drug given, and the method of administration all have an effect on absorption. Some drugs dissolve in the mouth and are absorbed into the bloodstream directly through the lining of the mouth. Some are swallowed and enter the bloodstream through the walls of

BEGINS	ROUTE	EXAMPLE
In the mouth	Sublingual	Nitroglycerin
In the stomach/intestine	Oral	Ibuprofen
In the muscle	IM	Meperidine
Under the skin	SC	Epinephrine, Insulin
In the bloodstream	IV	Antibiotics

the stomach or intestine. Drugs that are injected into skin or muscles pass into the bloodstream through nets of tiny blood vessels that nourish these areas.

Some drugs are not absorbed but are injected directly into the bloodstream. Drugs applied to the skin are usually intended not to be absorbed into the blood, but rather to affect only the cells in the skin layers.

The elderly tend not to have much difficulty with the process of absorption, but when they do, it may be due to a reduction of cells and their functions.

Distribution

After a drug is absorbed into the bloodstream, it is carried throughout the body by a complex network of blood vessels. Some of the drug passes out of the bloodstream through the thin walls of tiny vessels called **capillaries.** The drug then enters body cells through pores in the outer cell layers. It may also pass through cells into the fluid-filled spaces between the cells. This movement of the drug into the body cells and into the spaces between cells is called **distribution.** The exact path that any given drug follows depends on the interaction between the drug and specific body tissues. Some tissues can combine with certain drugs and others cannot.

Distribution is affected by the chemical makeup of the drug, the amount of drug given, and cell conditions such as temperature and pH. If distribution is slow, the effect of the drug is not felt until some time after administration. If distribution is fast, drug effects are noticed almost immediately after administration. Some drugs tend to collect in certain organs or tissues, called **reservoirs.** If drugs do collect in reservoirs, they are released into the body more slowly than drugs that are evenly distributed at the start.

For the elderly, the growth of adipose tissue may cause drug accumulation in these reservoirs.

Biotransformation

Metabolism or **biotransformation** is a series of chemical reactions that break down the drug into different substances that are easier for the body to eliminate. This is a natural process much like the digestion of food. It is necessary so that the body can rid itself of the waste products that are left over after the cells make use of nutrients or drugs.

Enzymes are special body proteins that speed up the process of biotransformation. They cause chemical reactions to occur thousands of times faster than they ordinarily would. Most of the biotransformation of drugs takes place in the liver. This very important organ, located in the abdominal cavity, is responsible for many body chemical reactions. Biotransformation also takes place to some extent in the lungs, the intestines, and the kidneys.

Some drugs cannot work on body cells until they are broken down chemically, so that biotransformation actually changes them into active drugs. Other drugs become inactive and lose their power to work on body cells when they are biotransformed. With some drugs this is good, because if these drugs were to remain unchanged in the body, they could collect and cause harm.

Some drugs do not need to be biotransformed in order to be eliminated. Ether, for example, passes out of the body in exactly the same chemical form as it entered. Its odor can be detected in the urine.

Here again, the elderly must be mentioned in regard to liver function. A decrease in size and function with age may interfere with the formation of body substances or enzymes necessary for biotransformation.

Excretion

Excretion is the body's way of removing the waste products of ordinary cell processes. Drugs are excreted in the same way as other waste products. Most drugs leave the body through the kidneys and the large intestine. In the kidneys, blood is filtered and liquid waste products collect in the form of urine. In the large intestine, undigested solid wastes collect in the form of feces.

Excretion also takes place in the lungs, where gaseous wastes, such as carbon dioxide and some types of drugs, are collected from the bloodstream. These are excreted when the person exhales. Anesthetic gases such as ether and chloroform are sometimes excreted through the lungs. Some drugs are excreted in the sweat and some even in hair. Milk glands also excrete some types of drugs. This is an important fact to know when giving medications to nursing mothers. Drugs that leave the body in a mother's milk may cause harm to the baby.

If a drug is excreted quickly, its effects are short-lived. If it is excreted slowly, its effects last longer. The rate of excretion depends on the chemical composition of the drug, the rate of biotransformation, and how often the drug is administered. The condition of the excreting organs will also determine how quickly and completely excretion takes place.

For example, in the elderly, more than 50 percent of the nephron units are nonfunctional. This reduces glomerular filtration by half. Reduced kidney function can also cause the problem of drug accumulation.

FACTORS AFFECTING DRUG ACTION

No two people are exactly alike, and no drug will affect every human body in exactly the same way. Body cells differ according to a person's age, size, sex, genetic inheritance, and physical and emotional condition. These personal characteristics may cause slightly different drug actions in different people given the same drug (Figure 2-4).

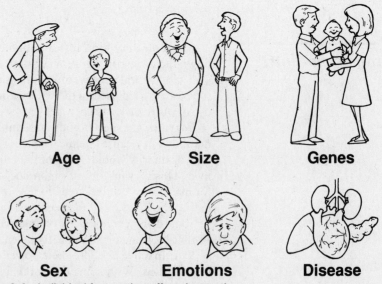

Age **Size** **Genes**

Sex **Emotions** **Disease**

Figure 2-4 Individual factors that affect drug action.

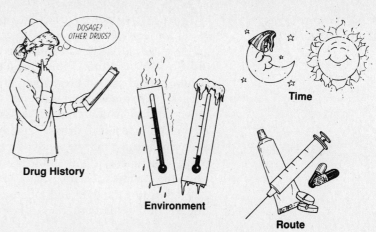

Figure 2-5 Administration factors that affect drug action.

Factors surrounding the administration of medications may also cause differences in people's responses to a drug. The route of administration, the time of day, the number and size of doses, and environmental conditions all play a role in drug action (Figure 2-5). Physicians take these factors into account before deciding which drug to prescribe and how much to prescribe.

Age

Most standard dosages are based on the amount of a drug that will cause the desired effect in an average adult. The bodies of very young and very old patients, however, do not function exactly like the average adult body.

In infants, the body systems are not fully developed. They may have trouble biotransforming or excreting drugs. Growing children must not take drugs that might affect their development. The body systems of the elderly may not function as efficiently as when they were middle-aged. The aging process slows down the work of certain organs, and older people are more prone to diseases that affect biotransformation and excretion. Therefore, smaller doses and different drugs are required in treating the young or the old.

Size

The size of a person and whether he or she is fat or lean have a bearing on drug action. An average dose given to a tall or obese person may have little effect. This is because there will be a low concentration of the drug in the bloodstream, body fluids, and cells. The same dose given to a small or thin person may cause too high a concentration of the drug in the body. The proper dose is usually worked out according to a formula that takes into account body weight, age, and/or the distribution of the drug.

It should be mentioned, though, that with age some tissue is replaced by adipose tissue, and this could cause a buildup of some medications such as barbiturates in the cells. Therefore, you must always be watchful of your patients' response to long-term barbiturate therapy and report any unusual actions by them.

Sex

The sex of a person may influence drug action. Women may react more strongly to certain drugs than men do. This is partly because of their generally smaller size and their higher proportion of body fat. Pregnant women must be extremely careful about taking any medication. Some drugs may harm the fetus.

Genetic Factors

The individual makeup of each person causes slight differences in basic processes like biotransformation, which then affects drug action. Some people have very unusual drug reactions that may be linked to genetic factors.

Disease Conditions

Diseases can strongly affect how patients respond to drugs. The organs necessary for biotransformation and excretion may be impaired. Diseases of the liver and kidneys especially will affect the processing and elimination of drugs. Heart disease, kidney failure, diabetes, and low blood pressure are disorders known to require special care in prescribing drugs. But any disease can change the effectiveness of a drug without warning.

Many older patients have diseases of both the liver and kidneys. Therefore, their responsiveness to drugs is greatly hindered. Often a drug cannot be used at all. Even though it may be specific for the patient's disease, the liver cannot change it to the therapeutically useful form, or elimination of the drug is impossible because the kidneys are damaged.

Cirrhosis of the liver and inflammation of the kidneys are two examples of diseases of the elderly that affect how patients respond to drugs.

Emotional Condition

The patient's mental state is an important factor in the success or failure of drug therapy. A patient with a positive attitude is likely to respond well to medication. A patient in a bad mood or in a state of depression or despair may not respond to some drugs. Strong feelings such as worry, jealousy, anger, or fear may have a noticeable effect on drug action.

Sometimes a positive drug effect occurs simply because the patient has taken something that is supposed to make him or her "feel better." This effect has nothing to do with the action of the drug itself. It is a psychological effect called the **placebo effect.** If the patient understands the disease and its treatment and has a positive attitude, the placebo effect can add to the effectiveness of medication therapy.

As a member of the health care team, you can do much to create a positive attitude in the patient. One way is to review the important reasons for taking the medication. Another is to treat the patient in a cheerful and caring manner. And, finally, your own positive, confident attitude toward the drugs you administer will influence the patient's response to medication.

Route of Administration

Drugs are absorbed, distributed, and biotransformed differently when given by different means or routes (see Chapter 3). This can affect drug action. A drug will act most quickly when injected directly into the bloodstream. Drugs injected into or under the skin or into muscles require more time to take effect. Medications administered by mouth take the longest time to show their effects.

Time of Day

Care must always be taken to give drugs at the time of day ordered by the physician. There are many time-related factors that influence drug action. Drugs taken by mouth are usually given between meals, when the patient has an empty stomach. However, certain stomach-irritating drugs may be taken with meals to avoid patient discomfort. When possible, drugs that make the patient sleepy are ordered to be taken at bedtime. Drugs with stimulating effects are given at times when they will not interfere with sleep. Normal bodily functions also vary with the time of day, thus affecting drug action.

Drug-Taking History

Drug action depends on whether a patient has previously taken doses of the same or another drug. Some drugs tend to collect in the body. In this case, later doses must be made smaller to avoid overmedicating the patient. Repeated doses of a drug may also make a patient less responsive to its effects. In that case, larger doses are required for the same effect.

Certain combinations of drugs can slow down or speed up effects, or they can cause unusual and sometimes dangerous reactions. This is why patients' medical histories and charts must include careful records of the drugs they have recently taken. Doctors should also check medical histories to find out whether patients are allergic to particular drugs such as penicillin.

This area can be a problem for the elderly. They often see several doctors who may be unaware of each other and of the other drugs being prescribed. Each doctor prescribes what is needed in a patient's particular case, unaware of the medications other doctors have prescribed. Multiple doctors and multiple drugs can lead to serious drug interactions. "Elder-Ed: Using Your Medicines Wisely: A Guide for the Elderly" is part of a model education program for the prevention of medication misuse by the elderly. This information can be helpful, especially if you work with the elderly at home. It is available from the National Institute on Drug Abuse, 5600 Fishers Lane, Rockville, MD 20857.

Environmental Conditions

Extremes of weather affect the action of drugs because body functions are influenced by heat and cold. Heat relaxes the blood vessels and speeds up the circulation, so drugs act faster. Cold slows their action by constricting the blood vessels and slowing the circulation. High altitude puts the body under stress because there is less oxygen in the air. This makes some drugs ineffective.

DRUG EFFECTS

The term **action** means the way the drug produces chemical changes in cells and tissues. The drug **effect** is the combination of biological and physical changes that take place in the body as a result of the drug action.

A drug is usually prescribed on the basis of its **main effect.** This is the desired therapeutic effect, or the reason the drug was administered. However, most drugs have additional effects on the body that are not part of the goal of drug therapy. These are called **side effects.**

A physician must always take possible side effects into account when planning drug treatment. Side effects can be harmless, mildly annoying, or dangerous. Sometimes unpleasant side effects are tolerated because of the therapeutic value of the main effect. For example, morphine is administered for its painkilling effect, but it also has the side effects of respiratory depression, constipation, and urine retention.

Many side effects can be controlled or lessened by using other drugs or special procedures. For example, aspirin, taken orally, is very beneficial for the treatment of arthritis but tends to irritate the lining of the stomach. This side effect is controlled by giving the drug with a glass of milk or with large amounts of water. To cite another example, diuretics can help ease water retention, but they may cause the body to excrete too much potassium. This situation can be corrected by giving potassium chloride or suggesting that the patient eat potassium-rich foods such as bananas.

A partial list of common side effects is presented in Table 2-1. The list is not for you to memorize but to show you the wide range of side effects that are possible. Side effects are related to the actions of specific drugs. In later chapters you will learn which side effects accompany which drugs.

Drug effects are classified as either local or systemic. Some drugs affect mainly the area where they enter or are applied to the body: for example, eyedrops, sunburn creams, suppositories, and throat lozenges. These drugs are given for their **local** effects. Other drugs travel through the bloodstream to affect cells or tissues in various parts of the body. These are given for their **systemic** effects.

Proper administration of medications requires both knowledge of drug effects and observation of the results in the patient. The prescribed dosage is the physician's best guess as to which drug and how much of the drug is needed to bring about the desired effect in a specific patient.

TABLE 2-1 Common Side Effects of Drugs

Anxiety	Insomnia
Black (tarry) stools	Irritability
Blurred vision	Itching
Breast tenderness	Lightheadedness
Breathing difficulties	Loss of appetite
Bruising	Low blood pressure
Burning sensation	Menstrual irregularities
Chest pains	Nasal stuffiness
Confusion	Nausea
Constipation	Nervousness
Cramps	Palpitations
Depression	Rash
Diarrhea	Restlessness
Dizziness	Ringing in the ears
Drowsiness	Sweating
Dryness of mouth, nose, skin	Tingling
Edema (swelling)	Tremors
Fatigue	Twitching
Fever	Upset stomach
Flushing	Urinary frequency
Headache	Urine discoloration
Heartburn	Urine retention
Hiccups	Vaginal discharge
Hives	Weakness
Impotence	Weight gain

When you give medications, consider whether the drug is given for a local or a systemic effect. Then, while observing the patient's reaction, determine whether you are seeing the drug's main effect or a side effect (Figure 2-6). Your knowledge of drug effects is important to the work of the entire health care team—and is especially important to your patient.

ADVERSE REACTIONS

With proper administration, a drug usually has the desired effect—the patient feels better, bodily functions are restored, and side effects are under control. However, occasionally the body will react to a drug in an unexpected way that may endanger the patient's health and safety. These unexpected conditions are called

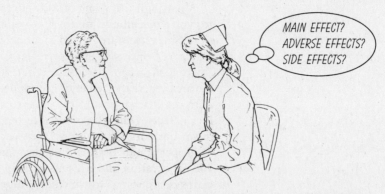

Figure 2-6 Questions to ask yourself while observing for medication effects.

adverse reactions. The most common adverse reactions will be described later, along with their causes, symptoms, and treatments.

As a person giving medications, you are expected to be aware of these possible reactions and notify your supervisor as soon as you notice any telltale signs. You may find it helpful to review this section again after studying the remaining chapters. By then you will have a better understanding of how these adverse reactions come about and how to recognize them.

Drug Allergy

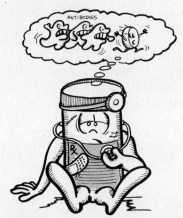

Figure 2-7 Drug allergy.

Drug allergy is an abnormal response that occurs because a person has developed **antibodies** against a particular drug (Figure 2-7). When a person takes the allergy-causing drug, called the **antigen,** the antibodies attack it. The reaction between antigen and antibodies causes damage to the body tissues. The injured cells release a substance called **histamine,** which is responsible for the symptoms usually seen in allergic reactions.

Mild allergic symptoms can occur immediately after the drug is taken, or they can show up hours, days, or even weeks later. Severe allergic reactions, which can be fatal, usually begin within minutes of exposure and may require immediate emergency treatment.

In drug references, you may read warnings about **drug hypersensitivity,** which is an allergic reaction that develops over time, for example, when a person is taking a course of antibiotics. When this occurs, the person must be switched to another drug.

To avoid the problem of drug allergy, physicians try to find out whether patients have a history of allergies, such as hay fever, asthma, or skin rashes. They also ask whether patients have shown unusual reactions to any drugs taken in the past.

◆ **DRUG ALLERGY** ◆ ◆ ◆ ◆ ◆ ◆ ◆ ◆ ◆ ◆ ◆ ◆ ◆

SYMPTOMS

• Mild: skin rashes, swelling or puffiness, nasal drainage, itchy eyes or skin, fever, and wheezing.

• Severe: shock reaction (called anaphylactic shock or anaphylaxis), shown by severe breathing problems (dyspnea), extreme weakness, nausea or vomiting, and a bluish color to the skin (cyanosis).

• Severe low blood pressure (hypotension) and stopping of the heart (cardiac arrest) can also develop.

TREATMENT

• Notify supervisor immediately and follow instructions.

• Emergency treatment will be required for anaphylactic shock and hypotension.

• Antihistamines, epinephrine, and drugs that relieve dyspnea may be ordered by a physician.

• For milder symptoms, similar drugs are used but in smaller doses, and the patient is advised to avoid the allergy-producing drug in the future. Skin tests may be ordered to pinpoint the source of the allergy.

Unusual Effect (Idiosyncrasy)

Some people have strange or unique responses to certain drugs (Figure 2-8). These unusual effects, or **idiosyncrasies,** are thought to be caused by genetic factors that change the way particular drugs are biotransformed.

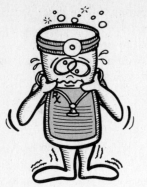

Figure 2-8 Unusual effect (idiosyncracy).

Tolerance

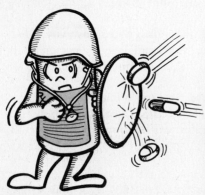

Figure 2-9 Tolerance.

Drug **tolerance** is resistance to the effect of a drug (Figure 2-9). The exact way in which tolerance develops is not yet understood. It is known to occur in some people after repeated dosages of the same or a similar drug. In order to get the full effect of the drug, those patients have to take increasingly larger doses.

Cumulation

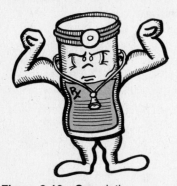

Figure 2-10 Cumulation.

Cumulation occurs when the body cannot biotransform and excrete one dose of a drug completely before the next dose is given (Figure 2-10). With repeated doses, the drug starts to collect in the blood and body tissues. This can be dangerous because high concentrations of many drugs are poisonous, or **toxic,** and can damage body cells.

Overdose and Toxicity

Through error, poor judgment, or attempted suicide, a patient may receive an overdose—a dose that is too large for his or her age, size, and/or physical condition. This can be dangerous because any drug can act like a poison if taken in too large a dose. Toxicity refers to the drug's ability to poison the body (Figure 2-11).

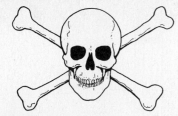

Figure 2-11 Toxicity.

Drug Interactions (Synergism and Antagonism)

Sometimes two or more drugs are given to a patient as part of drug therapy, or a patient may be taking an OTC medication at home for some other ailment. Whenever more than one drug is taken, the possibility of a drug interaction has to be considered. Two or more drugs may interact, with the result that the degrees and kinds of effects produced may be altered. This is called a drug interaction.

When two drugs administered together produce a more powerful response than the sum of their individual effects, this is called synergism or **potentiation** (Figure 2-12). Patients who take sedatives, for example, are advised to avoid drinking alcoholic beverages. This is because alcohol causes sedatives to have a much stronger, possibly fatal, effect. When two drugs interact to cause a lesser response than the sum of their individual effects, this is called **antagonism** (Figure 2-13, pg. 35). Antacids such as *Gelusil* should not be given to patients who are on oral tetracycline, an antibiotic, because they work against the absorption of tetracycline through the intestines.

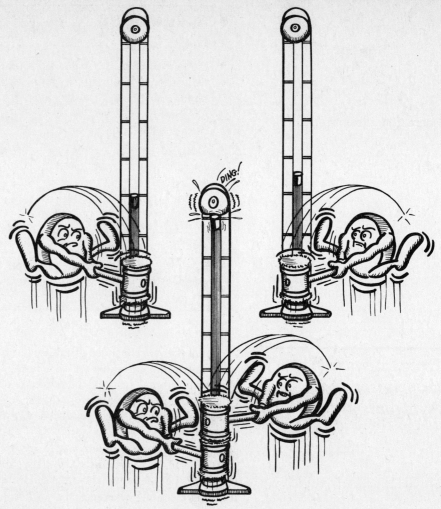

Figure 2-12 Synergism or potentiation (combined drug effects are more than individual effects).

Food can also affect drug absorption and can interact with drugs. Food–drug interactions can occur, and you should be aware of them.

There are many other ways in which drugs interact. Some of these interactions are bad, but not all. In fact, doctors sometimes make use of known drug interactions to control unwanted side effects or to increase the therapeutic effect of a particular drug. Probenecid is sometimes given with penicillin G. Probenecid slows the excretion of the antibiotic. This effect results in higher blood levels or allows a smaller dose of penicillin to be given.

It is the unplanned drug interactions that are of concern in administering medications. It takes the cooperation of every member of the health care team to guard against the administration of drugs that interact in unplanned ways.

Other Drug-Related Disorders

Some drugs, when administered over a period of time, can cause changes in body functioning or damage to certain organs. Bone marrow disease and a lower production of blood cells may result from fluorouracil therapy in cancer patients. Diseases of the liver and kidney may be caused by certain drugs. Drugs can also have negative effects on behavior and emotions. Antianxiety drugs such as *Valium* have been known to disturb sleep and cause nightmares. Irritability and nervousness are common problems with many drugs.

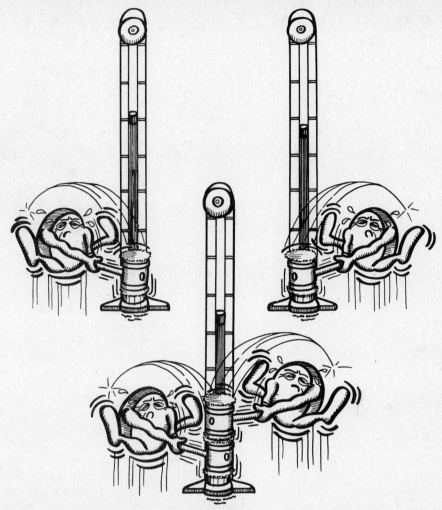

Figure 2-13 Antagonism (combined effects are less than the two individual effects).

Drug Dependence

Drug **dependence** is a strong psychological and/or physical need to take a certain drug (Figure 2-14). This need develops when a person takes a drug over a period of time. Usually the drug was prescribed to relieve pain or to control some physical or emotional problem. Eventually, some people find that they cannot seem to get along without the drug. They keep on taking it just to avoid the discomfort they would feel if they stopped.

Drug dependence can be either psychological or physical. In psychological or emotional dependence or **habituation,** a person has a drive or a craving to take a certain drug for pleasure or to relieve discomfort. There are no physical symptoms if the drug is taken away, but the person may feel anxious about not having the psychological crutch.

♦ **OTHER DRUG-RELATED DISORDERS** ♦

SYMPTOMS
- Depend on condition.

TREATMENT
- Report all suspicious symptoms and follow instructions.

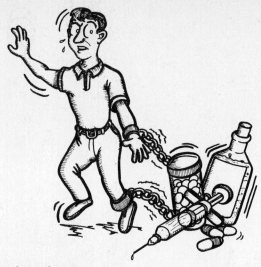

Figure 2-14 Drug dependence.

In physical dependence (also called addiction or chemical dependence), the body has grown so accustomed to the drug that it needs the drug in order to function. When the drug is taken away, the person develops **withdrawal symptoms** involving extreme physical discomfort. Eventually, if no further dose of the drug is administered, the body returns to normal functioning.

◆ **DRUG DEPENDENCE** ◆ ◆ ◆ ◆ ◆ ◆ ◆ ◆ ◆

SYMPTOMS

- Physical dependence: craving for a drug. If the drug is not administered, the patient develops symptoms of withdrawal, such as nausea, vomiting, tremors, sweating, and extreme physical discomfort.

- Psychological dependence: psychological craving for a drug. (This is present in physical dependence, too.) Patient displays anxiety and fear of physical discomfort when the drug is not administered.

TREATMENT

- Notify supervisor and follow instructions.

- With physical dependence, the physician may substitute another similar drug to ease the withdrawal symptoms and then gradually reduce the dosage of the substitute drug.

- With both physical and psychological dependence, counseling may be needed to help the patient get along without the drug.

- In the case of the dying or terminal patient who is in a great deal of pain, drug dependence may be allowed to develop so that the patient can be as comfortable as possible.

DRUG DEPENDENCE OR DRUG ABUSE?

Drug dependence is a problem any health care worker may have to deal with in giving medications. The time may come when a patient asks for more pain medication, for example, and you may be worried that the patient is becoming too dependent on the drug. Is this drug abuse?

In this situation, your main responsibility is to consult the nurse in charge. The decision on whether to medicate the patient further must be made jointly by the members of the health care team. Your own concerns may be eased, however, if you understand something about the difference between drug dependence and drug abuse.

Drug abuse usually refers to taking a certain drug not for medical reasons, but for the psychological or emotional effects it produces. Feelings of euphoria or calmness or a heightened awareness of the senses (feeling "high") are some of the reasons people take these drugs. Some experts define drug abuse as taking any drug to the point where it interferes with health and daily living patterns.

◆   **COMMONLY ABUSED DRUGS**   ◆ ◆ ◆ ◆ ◆ ◆

- narcotics and opium
- barbiturates ("downers"), sedatives or hypnotics, alcohol, and other depressants
- amphetamines, cocaine, and other stimulants ("uppers," "speed")
- LSD and other hallucinogens
- marijuana ("pot," "dope")
- anabolic steriods

Most of the commonly abused drugs are controlled substances, which you studied in Chapter 1. All of these drugs can create psychological dependence, and the barbiturates and narcotics can create physical dependence as well. However, drug abuse does not necessarily mean drug dependence.

Drug abuse is part of a larger and more widespread problem—**drug misuse** (Figure 2-15). This is overuse or careless use of any drug. Drug misuse is most often a problem with people who are taking their own medications at home. Tranquilizers, stimulants, and pain-killing drugs are frequently misused, and so are such common OTC drugs as laxatives. Nicotine and alcohol are widely misused, and both can create serious physical as well as psychological dependence. As you can see, there is little difference between drug abuse and drug misuse.

The important thing to remember is that both drug abuse and drug misuse endanger people's health and well-being. This includes the medical staff as well as patients. As a health care worker, you can help by keeping medicines locked up when not in use, administering only prescribed medications, and watching for signs of drug dependence and improper use of drugs.

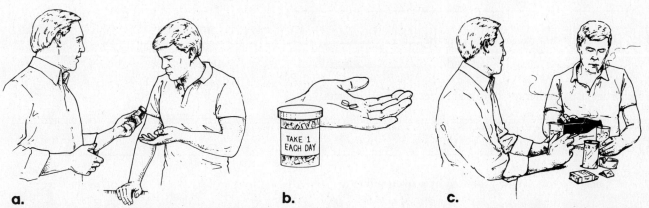

a.   **b.**   **c.**

Figure 2-15   a. Using someone else's prescription is dangerous; b. Follow directions—don't take more drug than prescribed; c. Nicotine and alcohol are drugs, too.

Using Medical Terminology

Complete the following statements.

1. The way a drug changes the chemistry of the body is called the drug _____

2. The physical changes that occur because of the drug action are called the drug _____

3. Absorption is _____
_____

4. Distribution is _____
_____

5. Biotransformation is _____
_____

6. Excretion is_____
_____

7. Drug effects that result from a drug circulating through the body are called _____ effects.

8. Drug effects that are confined to the area where the drug was administered are called _____ effects.

Acquiring Knowledge of Medications

Complete the following statements.

9. Drugs act by _____, _____, or _____ the work of the cells.

10. Drugs also act by _____ substances that the body fails to produce.

11. Drug action is affected by four bodily processes: _____, _____, _____, and _____

12. The organs that excrete waste are the _____, _____, _____, and _____

13. Drugs used in therapy have main effects and side effects.

    Main effects are _____

14. Side effects are _____

15. A placebo effect can be produced by a sugar pill or an
_____
_____

16. Drug abuse is _____

_____

17. Drug misuse is _____

_____

18. Withdrawal symptoms include _____

_____

19. Five groups of drugs that are often abused are _____

_____

20. If you suspect drug abuse, your obligation is to _____

_____

21. Physical drug dependence is _____

_____

22. Psychological drug dependence is _____

_____

Answer the following questions in the spaces provided.

23. What is the basis for treatment of drug overdose?

_____

_____

24. What treatment or approach is secondary?

_____

_____

25. How soon is a patient symptomatic of overdose?

_____

_____

26. What does alcohol do for a patient who has taken an overdose?

_____

_____

27. What is the approach to treatment if you do not know for sure but are told by the patient that he or she took an overdose?

_____

_____

28. Are central nervous system drugs the most sufficient supportive care for drug overdose? Explain.

_____

_____

_____

Applying Knowledge on the Job

The following is a list of patient characteristics. Place a check by those that you think might influence drug action.

_____ 29. Physical strength

_____ 30. Kidney disease

_____ 31. Deafness

_____ 32. Old age

_____ 33. Genes

_____ 34. Sex

_____ 35. Food likes and dislikes

_____ 36. Popularity

_____ 37. Infancy

_____ 38. Anger

_____ 39. Obesity

_____ 40. Poor circulation

_____ 41. Nervousness

_____ 42. Tallness

_____ 43. Cheerful mood

_____ 44. Political affiliation

_____ 45. Drug-taking history

_____ 46. Hair color

_____ 47. Oral hygiene

Select the term that best completes each sentence and write it in the blank.

| antagonism | drug dependence | potentiation | cumulation | toxicity |
| drug allergy | drug interaction | tolerance | idiosyncrasy | |

48. After taking several doses of medicine, little Billy no longer seems to be affected by the drug. This may be a symptom of _____

49. Mrs. Jones gets a stronger drug effect with each additional dose of her medication. She may be showing signs of

_____

50. Two drugs producing a greater effect than the sum of their individual effects is referred to as

_____

51. The doctor has just canceled Ms. Williams' order for a sedative that helped her sleep after her operation. As the medication hour approaches, Ms. Williams expresses the worry that she will not be able to sleep without her medication. You see this as a possible sign of _____

52. Two drugs interacting to produce a lesser effect than the sum of the individual effects is called

_____

53. Annie Peterson is reacting in a peculiar way to her medication. You have never seen a person react this way to the medication she is taking. Drug allergy has been ruled out. Annie's response to the drug will probably be classified as a(n) _____

54. An adverse reaction resulting from an antibody attacking an antigen is called a(n) _____

55. You have recently given Mr. Smith a medication ordered by his doctor. Mr. Smith is not reacting to the drug the way you expected. In talking with him, you discover that he has also been taking medication he brought with him from home. You suspect that his adverse reaction is due to a(n) _____

56. Miss Grimes seems very sleepy and confused after receiving her medication. You check her records and discover

that someone misread the doctor's order and gave Miss Grimes a dose that was much too large. You notify the supervisor immediately because you think Miss Grimes is showing signs of _____

Using Resources on the Job

Obtain a current copy of the PDR from your school, nursing unit, or clinic. Use it to answer the following questions.

57. Name the form printed in the PDR that the FDA and pharmaceutical manufacturers encourage health care professionals to fill out and send to the FDA's Division of Epidemiology and Surveillance.

   _____

   _____

58. Where do you get this form?

   _____

   _____

59. What does (VAERS) signify? _____

   _____

   _____

60. Why should the physician refer to the contraindication section of the PDR or the manufacturer's package insert for each vaccine?

   _____

   _____

➤ ANSWERS TO CHAPTER 2 REVIEW ⬅

Using Medical Terminology

1. action

2. effects

3. passage of a substance into the bloodstream from the site of administration

4. movement of drugs into cells and into spaces between cells

5. breaking down drugs into different substances that can be excreted

6. removal of waste products from the body

7. systemic

8. local

Acquiring Knowledge of Medications

9. speeding up (stimulating), slowing down (depressing), stopping or destroying

10. replacing

11. absorption, distribution, biotransformation, excretion

12. kidneys, large intestine, lungs, milk glands

13. desired therapeutic effects; the reason the drug is given

14. other effects besides the desired therapeutic effect

15. infection of sterile water

16. using a drug for other than medical reasons or in such a way that it interferes with daily life

17. overuse or improper use of any drug

18. nausea, vomiting, tremors, sweating, and extreme physical discomfort

19. Any five of the following are correct: Narcotics and opium; barbiturates, sedatives or hypnotics, and alcohol; amphetamines, cocaine, and other stimulants; LSD and other hallucinogens; marijuana

20. consult the nurse in charge

21. a condition in which the body must have a drug in

order to function because it is so used to having the drug

22. a feeling of being unable to get along without a drug

23. symptomatic and supportive

24. gastric lavage, administration of specific drugs (i.e., antagonists, peritoneal or extracorporeal dialysis, forced diuresis)

25. usually 30 minutes to 2 hours

26. shortens the time needed for symptoms to appear

27. administer 100 g of activated charcoal powder in water

28. no; they are unnecessary drugs because they can cause other problems such as convulsions

Applying Knowledge on the Job

29. —

30. ✓

31. —

32. ✓

33. ✓

34. ✓

35. —

36. —

37. ✓

38. ✓

39. ✓

40. ✓

41. ✓

42. ✓

43. ✓

44. —

45. ✓

46. —

47. —

48. tolerance

49. cumulation

50. potentiation (or synergism)

51. drug dependence

52. antagonism

53. unusual effect (or idiosyncrasy)

54. drug allergy

55. drug interaction

56. toxicity

Using Resources on the Job

57. Adverse Event Report

58. in back of PDR and is allowed to be copied

59. Vaccine Adverse Event Reporting System

60. to compare it with the patient's history and the conditions at hand

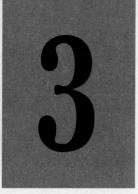

C
H
A
P
T
E
R

3

Fundamentals of Medication Therapy

◆◆ In this chapter you will learn about various forms of medications and the routes by which they are given. You will learn how to translate medication orders so that you can give medications in the proper form at the correct time and by the right route.

COMPETENCIES

After studying this chapter, you should be able to

- list the various forms of medication, ranging from liquids to solids.
- follow correct procedures for storing and using tinctures, fluidextracts, elixirs, spirits, and suspensions.
- tell how lotions, liniments, and ointments should be applied.
- explain what delayed-release tablets and capsules are and how they should be given to patients.
- state the rule for giving enteric-coated tablets and capsules.
- list and describe the routes for administering medications.
- tell who is allowed to give medications by the parenteral route.
- give the meanings of abbreviations for medication forms, routes, administration times, and general medical abbreviations.
- use the 24-hour clock.
- tell the difference between a physician's order sheet and a prescription blank.
- name the parts of a medication order.
- translate physician's orders into plain English.
- explain what to do if you cannot read or do not understand a medication order.

active ingredient: the ingredient in a product that produces the therapeutic effect

automatic stop order (ASO): same as self-terminating order

concentration: amount of drug in a certain amount of liquid

counterirritant: a drug that irritates tissues so as to relieve some other problem

enteric coated: coated with a substance that dissolves in the intestine but not in the stomach (enteric—pertaining to the small intestine)

infusion: placing a tube into a vein for the purpose of slowly adding fluids to the body (e.g., dextrose, plasma); also called intravenous (IV) drip

inhalation: administering drugs by way of droplets or mist that is breathed in

insertion: placing an object into a body cavity (e.g., putting a suppository into the rectum)

instillation: placing drops of liquid into the eyes, ears, nose, or some other body cavity

insufflation: blowing a powder into a body cavity

irrigation: rinsing a body cavity with water or other solutions

mucous membrane: moist, glossy lining of tubes inside the body (e.g., mouth, sinuses, rectum) that lets some liquids pass through into the body tissues

outpatient: patient who is not hospitalized or institutionalized; a walk-in (or ambulatory) patient

paste: stiff, thick ointment

physician's order sheet: a form for writing medication orders, located in the patient chart

preparation: the form in which a drug is made; either a liquid, solid, or something in between

scored: tablets with one or more grooves down the middle for ease in breaking the tablets into halves or quarters

self-terminating order: drug order that stops at a certain time or after a certain number of doses; also called automatic stop order

soluble: capable of being dissolved

solution: a liquid containing a dissolved drug

standing order: drug order that is to be continued until further notice

stat order: drug order carried out immediately and only once

sterile: germ free

suspension: a liquid containing undissolved particles of a drug

FORMS OF MEDICATION

Drugs are mixed with various ingredients to make them suitable for patients to take. There are ingredients to make oral medicines taste good. Old as well as young patients will take these medications better. There are ingredients to thin out a drug mixture so that the dosage can be controlled. Other ingredients allow drugs to be applied on the skin or placed into body parts such as the eyes, ears, or rectum. These combinations of drugs with various ingredients are called drug preparations or products.

Different forms of drugs are appropriate for different routes of administration, so it is very important to use the correct form. Failure to administer the drug in the correct form will result in medication error. Using an incorrect form also can cause damage to body cells. Therefore, you will need to learn something

TABLE 3-1: Abbreviations for Medication Forms

ABBREVIATION	FORM
cap., caps.	capsule
elix.	elixir
ext.	extract
fld. ext.	fluidextract
oint., ung.	ointment (unguent)
soln.	solution
sp.	spirit
supp.	suppository
syr.	syrup
tab.	tablet
tinct., tr.	tincture

about the various drug preparations and their uses. You should memorize the abbreviations given in Table 3-1.

Medication forms are loosely classified as either liquids or solids. But many forms are closer to semiliquids or semisolids. Other medications are gases (e.g., anesthetic agents and amyl nitrite).

Liquids and Semiliquids

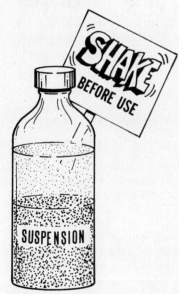

Figure 3-1 Shake suspension before use.

Many drugs are administered in liquid form. They may be given by mouth, rubbed onto the skin, or dropped into eyes, ears, or other parts of the body. Liquid preparations are useful because they allow rapid absorption of the drug. For children and elderly patients who have trouble swallowing solid capsules or tablets, liquid oral medicines are especially helpful.

Some drugs are able to dissolve in liquids, and others are not. When **active ingredients** are mixed with water, alcohol, or both, the resulting preparations are either solutions or suspensions. In **solutions,** the drug is dissolved in the alcohol or water. In **suspensions,** the drug is not dissolved, but tiny particles or droplets of the drug are held, or suspended, in an even distribution throughout the liquid.

In suspensions that are left standing for a while, particles settle to the bottom of the bottle (oils rise to the top). The clear liquid portion is then visible. This situation is normal and can be corrected by shaking the bottle well before giving the medication (Figure 3-1). Solutions, on the other hand, rarely separate when left standing. If they do, it is because they have been stored improperly. Separated solutions must be discarded.

Within the broad categories of solutions and suspensions, there are several specific liquid forms of medication. These are described below. Tinctures, fluidextracts, elixirs, spirits, and syrups are all types of solutions. Emulsions, magmas, gels, and lotions are types of suspensions.

Tinctures. Tinctures are solutions made with alcohol or alcohol with water. The active ingredients make up 10–20% of the solution. Examples are tincture of iodine, belladonna tincture, paregoric, and Tincture of Merthiolate.

Fluidextracts. Fluidextracts are very concentrated alcohol solutions that contain drugs from plant sources.

Elixirs. Elixirs are solutions of alcohol and water containing 10–20% of a drug. Elixirs have special added ingredients to make them sweet-tasting and pleasant-smelling. They are often used as oral medications for children and the elderly. Phenobarbital elixir and *Benadryl* elixir are examples.

Chapter 3 Fundamentals of Medication Therapy **45**

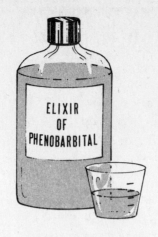

Keep tightly capped

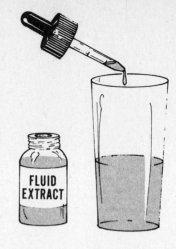

Small doses — measure carefully

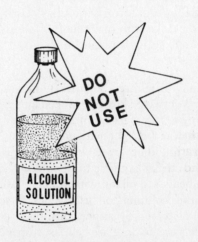

Do not use if separated

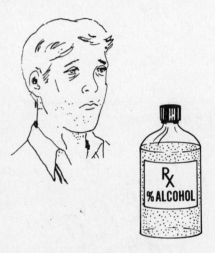

Not for alcoholics

Figure 3-2   Rules for alcohol solutions.

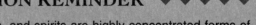

◆   **ADMINISTRATION REMINDER**   ◆ ◆ ◆ ◆ ◆

Tinctures, fluidextracts, elixirs, and spirits are highly concentrated forms of drugs (Figure 3-2). They contain much higher amounts of drug per unit of liquid than do other liquid forms. These preparations must be measured very carefully, using a dropper or a medicine glass. The medicine may be added to water, juice, or another solution suggested by the doctor. The patient then drinks this mixture.

Caution: Tinctures, fluidextracts, elixirs, and spirits contain alcohol. Do not administer to a diagnosed alcoholic. Storage is very important with these alcohol solutions. They must be kept tightly stoppered so that the alcohol cannot evaporate. Store them in a dark place, as stated on labels. Otherwise, the drug may separate out from the alcohol. If this should happen, do not use the preparation but order another.

Spirits. Spirits are alcohol solutions of volatile oils, or oils that evaporate. For example, camphor oil mixed with alcohol is called camphor spirit. Spirits contain 5–20% active ingredients.

Syrups. Syrups are heavy solutions of water and sugar, usually with a flavoring added. They are mixed with a very small amount of a drug. Syrups are useful for masking the bitter taste of certain drugs (e.g., orange and cherry syrups).

Emulsions. Emulsions are suspensions of oils and fats in water. Cod liver oil emulsion is an example.

Magmas. A magma contains heavy particles mixed with water that forms a milky liquid or paste. Milk of magnesia is a familiar example of a magma.

Gels. Gels are similar to magmas, but they contain finer particles.

◆ **ADMINISTRATION REMINDER** ◆ ◆ ◆ ◆ ◆

Emulsions, magmas, and gels are given in very small amounts because they contain large portions of active drug ingredients. Since they are suspensions, they must be shaken before use.

Liniments. Liniments are mixtures of drugs with water, alcohol, oil, or soap for external use. Liniments are rubbed onto the skin to promote absorption. They are used as soothing preparations or as counterirritants (drugs that mask pain in nearby muscles or skin by creating a different kind of irritation).

Lotions. Lotions are suspensions of drugs in a water base for external use. Lotions are patted onto the skin rather than being rubbed in (Figure 3-3). Lotions tend to settle out and must be shaken well before use. Calamine lotion is a com-

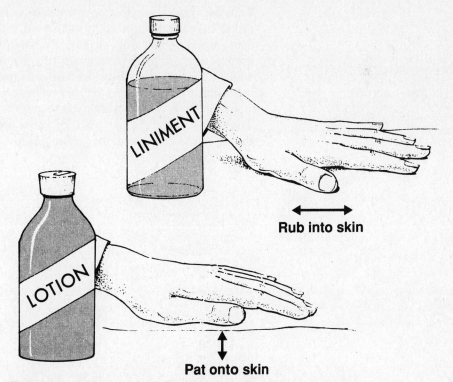

Rub into skin

Pat onto skin

Figure 3-3   Liniments and lotions are applied by different methods.

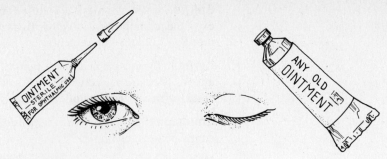

Figure 3-4 Ointments for the eyes are specially labeled.

mon example. Lotions have many uses: to protect, cool, lubricate, cleanse, or stimulate the skin.

Ointments. Ointments are drugs mixed in lanolin, a fine oil taken from the skin of the sheep, or in petrolatum, a jelly made from petroleum. They are usually applied to skin surfaces, but some ointments can be placed into the eyes. Eye ointments must always bear the label "Sterile—for ophthalmic use" (Figure 3-4). Thick, stiff ointments that do not melt at body temperature are called **pastes.**

Sprays. Liquid medications are sometimes prepared as sprays for application to the skin or mucous membranes. A special device sprays small droplets evenly across the surface to be medicated. Some sprays may be inhaled into the lungs.

Solids and Semisolids

Solid forms of drugs are widely used in drug treatment (Figure 3-5). There is no mixing, shaking, and measuring to be done, as there is with many liquids. The solid forms are also a convenient way to take unpleasant-tasting or irritating drugs.

Powders. Powders are fine, dry particles of drugs. They may be dissolved in liquids or used as is, depending on the physician's orders. Powders have both internal and external uses.

Tablets. Tablets are drug powders that have been pressed or molded into small disks. They are designed to be swallowed, either alone or with a liquid. Tablets come in a variety of sizes, shapes, and weights. Some have colored coatings, flavorings, and printed labels showing the manufacturer. Many tablets are **scored,** which means that they have one or more grooves down the middle. These make it possible to break the tablets into halves or quarters if needed.

Capsules. A capsule is a gelatin sheath that contains one dose of medication. The drug inside the capsule can be either a powder, an oil, or a liquid. When the capsule is swallowed, the gelatin quickly dissolves and releases the medicine into the stomach.

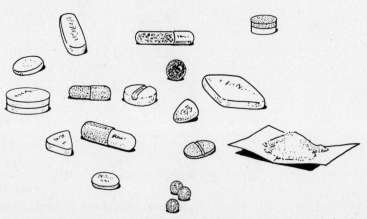

Figure 3-5 Solid forms of medication come in many shapes, sizes, and colors.

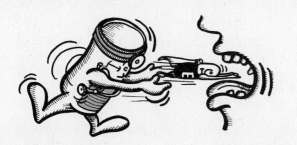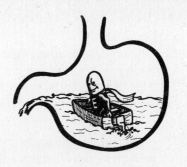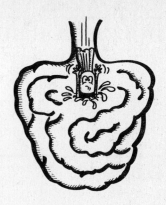

Figure 3-6   Enteric coating dissolves in the intestine.

Many different types of capsules are available. They come with hard or soft coverings in various sizes ranging from 7/16ths of an inch to 1 inch. Many of them have special shapes and colorings that indicate which company produced them.

Delayed-Release Tablets and Capsules. These forms contain several doses of a drug. The doses have special coatings that dissolve at different rates, so that medicine is released into the stomach gradually. Some doses are released immediately. Others are released up to 12 hours later. Delayed-release tablets and capsules allow for drug effects to continue at the same level over a long period of time. Sustained release and timed release are other terms used to describe these products.

Caution: Never crush, open, or empty a delayed-release tablet or capsule into food or liquid. Such actions could cause the patient to receive an overdose.

Enteric-Coated Tablets and Capsules. These are tablets and capsules with a special coating that keeps them from dissolving in the stomach (Figure 3-6). They do not dissolve until they reach the intestine. The **enteric coating** prevents an irritating drug from upsetting the stomach. It also prevents the stomach juices from interacting with the drug to change its effect.

◆   **ADMINISTRATION REMINDER**   ◆ ◆ ◆ ◆ ◆

If the patient is taking an enteric-coated product, watch carefully to see that the drug is taking effect. Some patients' intestines are not able to dissolve the enteric coating. Also, enteric-coated tablets and capsules must not be crushed or mixed into food or liquid. This would destroy the enteric coating and cause the medication to be released in the stomach instead of the intestine.

Troches and Lozenges. Troches and lozenges are tablets designed to dissolve in the mouth rather than being swallowed. They may be flat, round, or rectangular and are used for their local effects. As they dissolve, they bring a high concentration of drug into contact with the mouth and throat. They can help to relieve pain or soothe irritation in those areas.

Suppositories. Suppositories are drugs mixed with a firm substance that melts at body temperature. The drug mixture is molded into a shape suitable for insertion into the vagina, rectum, or urethra. After insertion, the suppository dissolves against the warm mucous membranes of these openings and releases the drug. The active ingredients take effect locally or are absorbed into the bloodstream for systemic effects.

ROUTES OF ADMINISTRATION

Drugs can be administered to patients through several methods or routes. Each route has its advantages and disadvantages. The route chosen will depend on the type of medication, the dosage form, and the desired effects. Abbreviations for routes of administration that you should know are given in Table 3-2.

Oral

In oral administration, a drug is given by mouth and swallowed, either alone or with a glass of liquid. The drug is then absorbed into the bloodstream through the lining of the stomach and intestine.

Oral administration is the easiest, safest, and most economical way for a patient to take medicine. However, it is also the slowest way for a drug to reach the cells of the body. The drug can be broken down by enzymes in the digestive system. Its absorption can be affected by the presence of food. Irritating medicines may cause nausea and stomach discomfort. Nevertheless, the oral route is well accepted and often used in drug therapy. Oral medications are usually in liquid, tablet, or capsule form.

Sublingual

Sublingual administration means placing a drug under the tongue, where it dissolves in the patient's saliva. It is quickly absorbed through the mucous membrane that makes up the lining of the mouth. The patient is not permitted to drink or eat until all of the medication is dissolved.

Compared to the oral route, the sublingual route has the advantage of more rapid absorption. It also yields a higher concentration of the drug in the blood, because the drug does not have to pass through the digestive system first. This is a convenient route as long as drugs are not irritating or bad-tasting.

Medications for sublingual administration are in the form of tablets. They are usually given for their systemic effects. Nitroglycerin, a drug that dilates heart vessels, is often administered sublingually. Ergotamine tartrate *(Ergostat)* may be given sublingually for migraine headache.

Buccal

Buccal administration is similar to sublingual administration except that the medication is placed in the mouth next to the cheek. The drug is absorbed through the mucous membrane that lines the inside of the cheek. Buccal medications are in the form of tablets. These should not be swallowed, and no food or drink is permitted until they are dissolved. Oxytocin, a drug that brings on labor in pregnant women, may be administered buccally.

TABLE 3-2:   Abbreviations for Routes

ABBREVIATION	ROUTE	MEANING
buc	buccal	inside the cheek
hypo, h, H, (h)	hypodermic	under the skin (same as subcutaneous)
ID	intradermal	into the skin
IM	intramuscular	into the muscle
IV	intravenous	into the vein
PO, p.o., O., o	oral	by mouth
p.r., r, R, IR	rectal/intrarectal	by rectum
p.v.	vaginal	by vagina
SC, sub-Q, SQ, subcu	subcutaneous	under the skin (into fatty layer)
subling, subl, SL	sublingual	under the tongue

Topical

Topical administration is the method of applying a drug directly to the skin or mucous membrane, usually for a local effect. Drugs for topical use are often designed to soothe irritated tissues or to prevent or cure local infections. They are in the form of creams, liniments, lotions, ointments, liquids, and powders. Liquids may be sprayed, swabbed, or painted onto the desired surfaces. Powders may be blown onto the skin or into body cavities (**insufflation**). Other forms are rubbed or patted on or held against skin surfaces with a bandage. Absorption through the skin is slow, while absorption through mucous membranes is rapid.

Topical medications can be dropped into the eyes, ears, and nose (**instillation**), and they can be inserted into the vagina, urethra, urinary bladder, and rectum (**insertion**). Any of these areas may also be rinsed with water containing drugs (**irrigation**). These applications are very easy to perform, but correct procedure must be followed to avoid damaging the tissue.

Rectal

Inserting medication into the rectum in the form of a suppository is called rectal administration. Enemas also are administered into the rectum. Absorption through the lining of the rectum is slow and irregular. However, this may be the best route when a patient cannot take medications orally. For example, a vomiting patient or an unconscious patient may require rectal administration.

Vaginal

The vaginal route of administration requires inserting a cream, foam, tablet, or suppository into the vagina. Medications inserted vaginally are usually given for their local effects, as in the treatment of a vaginal infection with *Mycostatin*.

Inhalation

In **inhalation** administration, medicine is sprayed or inhaled into the nose, throat, and lungs. The drug is absorbed through the mucous membranes in the nose and throat or through the tiny air sacs that fill the lungs. Drugs to be inhaled are in the form of gases or fine droplets (sprays, mists, steam, etc.)

The lungs contain a large surface area, so there is good absorption. However, it is hard to regulate the dose. The inhalation method is also awkward and not suitable for drugs that might irritate the lungs.

Inhalation is widely used for the rapid treatment of asthma symptoms. Special devices (e.g., inhalers, nebulizers, atomizers) are available that make inhalation therapy more convenient than in the past. Because germs can easily enter the body through the linings of the lungs, the equipment used for inhalation therapy must be very clean.

Parenteral

Parenteral administration involves injecting a drug into the body with a needle and syringe. This method gives much more rapid absorption and distribution than does oral administration. The dosage can also be controlled very carefully. The parenteral route is especially useful in emergencies, when a drug effect is needed immediately.

There are several disadvantages to the parenteral route. All injection equipment and medicines must be **sterile,** or free of germs. The method is expensive, sometimes painful, and not easy for patients to administer to themselves. Most

---

◆ **CAUTION** ◆ ◆ ◆ ◆ ◆ ◆ ◆ ◆ ◆ ◆ ◆ ◆ ◆ ◆ ◆

Parenteral administration requires special training, special safety precautions, and special equipment. State regulations allow only certain licensed health workers to administer medications parenterally: for instance, nurses.

important, there is the danger of injecting a drug incorrectly into a vein, which could cause serious harm and even death.

Medicine for injection must be in liquid form. Often it must be prepared as a suspension of a powder in distilled water.

The parenteral route is divided into four main categories, according to where the injection is given.

In intradermal (intracutaneous) administration, a small amount of medicine is injected just beneath the outer layer of skin. The dose is usually less than 0.3 ml. The injected drug forms a small bubble (bleb) under the skin. Intradermal injections are used in tuberculin tests, allergy tests, and vaccinations. The drug is absorbed very slowly in this type of injection.

In the subcutaneous route, medication is injected into a layer of fatty tissue that lies right below the skin. This is called the subcutaneous (under the skin) tissue. The dose is approximately 1–2 ml. Insulin, hormones, and local anesthetics are among the medications administered by subcutaneous injection.

Intramuscular administration is the injection of drugs deep into the muscles. Because the muscles are well supplied with blood, absorption from the muscles is faster than absorption from the skin layers. Muscles can also absorb a greater amount of fluid without discomfort to the patient; the usual dose is 1–3 ml. Intramuscular injection is also preferred for substances that would irritate the skin layers. Penicillin is often injected in this manner. During intramuscular administration, care must be taken to inject only large, healthy muscles and to avoid hitting major nerves, bones, and blood vessels.

In intravenous injection, a sterile drug solution is placed directly into a vein. This is the least safe method, but it may be necessary when medication is needed quickly. Dosages vary according to the situation.

Intravenous injection differs from intravenous infusion, or IV drip, mainly in speed of action. **Infusion** is the insertion of a tube or a needle into a vein through which fluids are slowly added to the bloodstream over a period of time. Infusion is used often in nursing care to keep the body's fluid level in balance. Drugs can be added to IV fluids for a continuous drug effect. Or they can be injected into the IV tube that leads into the vein, which is almost the same as injecting directly into the vein.

They may also be added via a volume-controlled chamber, heparin lock, special entry areas in an IV line, piggyback, or by a patient-controlled analgesic (PCA) pump.

Intracardiac, intra-arterial, intrathecal or intraspinal, and intraosseous are types of injections that only physicians are permitted to perform. In these methods, a drug is injected into the heart muscle, into an artery, into the spinal spaces, or into a bone, respectively.

THE MEDICATION ORDER

When a physician tells a nurse or another health care worker which drug or drugs to administer to a patient, the physician is giving a medication order. It may be expressed in writing or verbally.

Written orders are stated in a special book for doctors' orders or on a **physician's order sheet** in a patient's chart (Figure 3-7).

A prescription blank is used to write medication orders for patients who are being discharged from the hospital or who are seeing the doctor in a clinic (Figure 3-8). These patients are called **outpatients.**

Orders may be given verbally in an emergency when there is no time to write them down, or verbal orders may be given over the phone when the doctor is

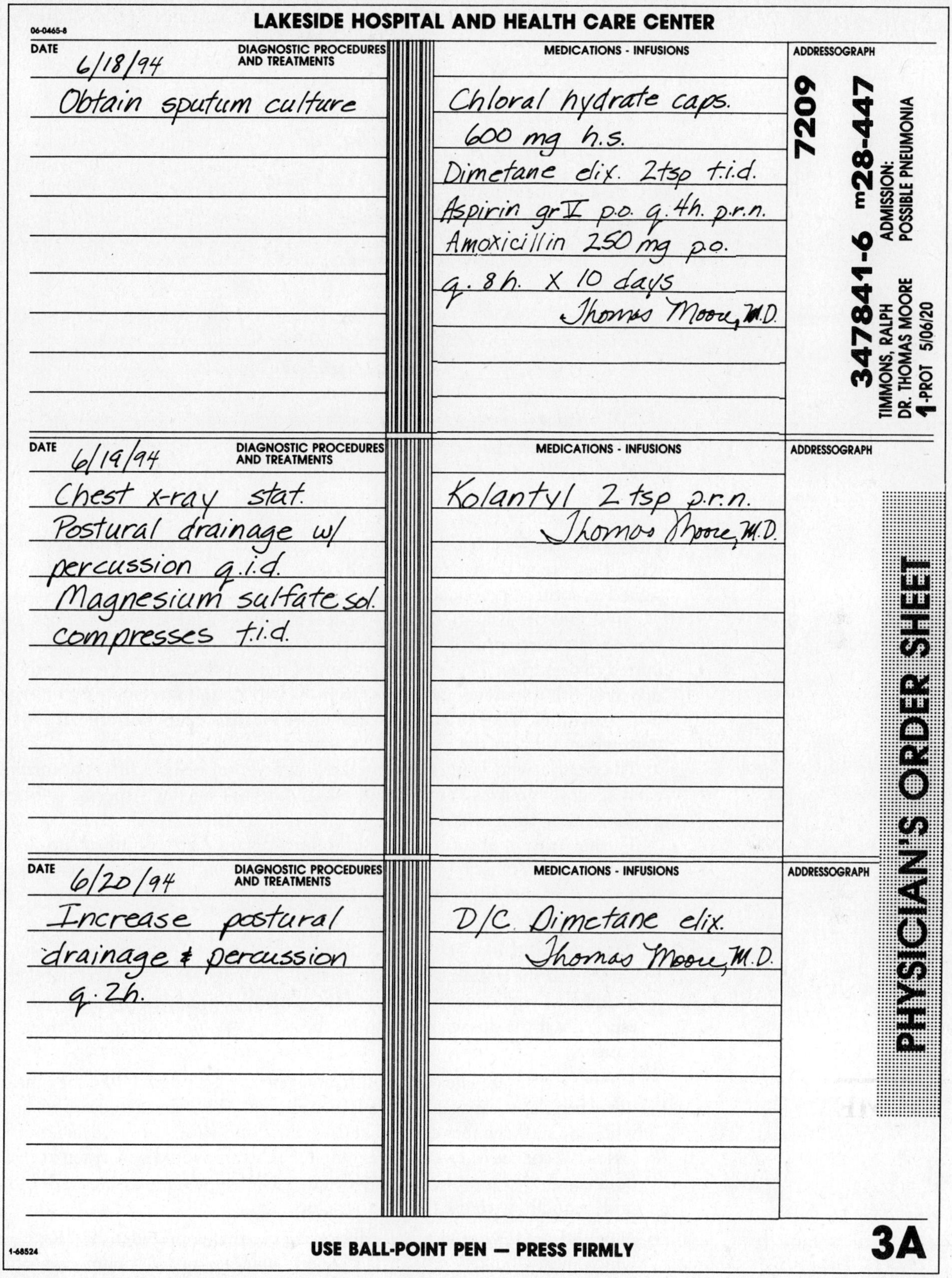

LAKESIDE HOSPITAL AND HEALTH CARE CENTER

06-0465-8

DATE 6/18/94	DIAGNOSTIC PROCEDURES AND TREATMENTS	MEDICATIONS - INFUSIONS	ADDRESSOGRAPH

Obtain sputum culture

Chloral hydrate caps.
600 mg h.s.
Dimetane elix. 2 tsp t.i.d.
Aspirin gr V p.o. q. 4h. p.r.n.
Amoxicillin 250 mg p.o.
q. 8h. X 10 days
　　　　　Thomas Moore, M.D.

7209　m28-447
347841-6
TIMMONS, RALPH
DR. THOMAS MOORE
1-PROT 5/06/20
ADMISSION:
POSSIBLE PNEUMONIA

DATE 6/19/94	DIAGNOSTIC PROCEDURES AND TREATMENTS	MEDICATIONS - INFUSIONS	ADDRESSOGRAPH

Chest x-ray stat.
Postural drainage w/
percussion q.i.d.
Magnesium sulfate sol.
compresses t.i.d.

Kolantyl 2 tsp p.r.n.
　　　Thomas Moore, M.D.

DATE 6/20/94	DIAGNOSTIC PROCEDURES AND TREATMENTS	MEDICATIONS - INFUSIONS	ADDRESSOGRAPH

Increase postural
drainage & percussion
q. 2h.

D/C. Dimetane elix.
　　　Thomas Moore, M.D.

PHYSICIAN'S ORDER SHEET

1-68524

USE BALL-POINT PEN — PRESS FIRMLY

3A

Figure 3-7 Physician's order sheet.

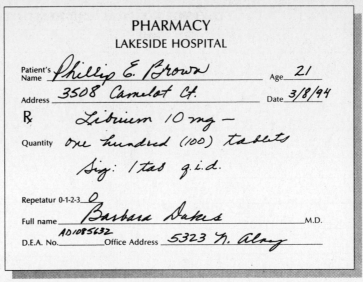

PHARMACY
LAKESIDE HOSPITAL

Patient's Name *Phillip E. Brown*   Age *21*

Address *3508 Camelot Ct.*   Date *3/8/94*

℞   *Librium 10 mg —*

Quantity *one hundred (100) tablets*

     Sig: 1 tab q.i.d.

Repetatur 0-1-2-3 *0*

Full name *Barbara Oakes*   M.D.

D.E.A. No. *AD1085632*   Office Address *5323 N. Alay*

Figure 3-8 Prescription blank for an outpatient.

away from the health facility. Some doctors routinely give verbal orders even when they are at the facility. In each case, the verbal order is written down and signed as soon as practical.

Physicians are usually the only people allowed to prescribe medicines, but in some states nurse practitioners, pharmacists, and physician's assistants are permitted to prescribe. These new members of the health care team frequently practice in health maintenance organizations (HMOs) and free-standing emergency health facilities. They prescribe drugs under the direct supervision of a physician with whom they work.

The person who is allowed to take down verbal orders differs according to each agency's policies. You should ask about your agency's specific policies regarding the writing and receiving of medication orders.

The medication order includes several important pieces of information. All of this information must be read and understood by you, the health care worker, so that you may correctly prepare and administer the medication. The basic parts of a medication order are as follows:

- *Patient's full name.* For proper identification, the patient's first and last names and the middle initial are needed. The patient's admission number is included in some health facilities. The patient's age should be included, especially if the dosage needs to be checked (e.g., for children and elderly patients).

- *Date of the order.* The day, month, and year are included. Often the time of day when the order was written is also shown. This helps avoid confusion when the staff changes shifts. The 24-hour clock is used in some facilities to lessen the chance of error. For example, 9:15 a.m. would be written as 0915 hours, and 5:45 p.m. would be written as 1745 hours. Study Figure 3-9 to understand how to use the 24-hour clock.

- *Name of the drug.* On a prescription blank, this is preceded by "Rx," which means "take." The drug's generic name or product name is written out. For reasons of cost, it is becoming more common for doctors to order drugs by their generic names. There may be a special line on the prescription blank for writing in the generic name or one that says "may substitute generic drug." If a drug name is not familiar to you, consult a drug reference such as the USP Drug Information for the Health Care Professional or the PDR.

THE 24 - HOUR CLOCK

When using the 24-hour clock, time is given in four digits. The first two digits stand for hours. The second two digits stand for minutes. The day begins at 0001 (12:01 am) and ends at 2400 hours (12:00 midnight).

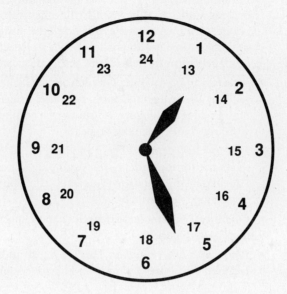

In the clock shown above, the am hours are numbered on the outer circle, as on regular clocks. The pm hours are numbered on the inner circle. These numbers are used after 1:00 pm. The hour 12:59 pm is expressed as 1259, and 1:00 pm is expressed as 1300 (thirteen-hundred hours). Note that no punctuation marks are used.

SAMPLE CONVERSIONS

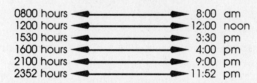

0800 hours	⟷	8:00 am
1200 hours	⟷	12:00 noon
1530 hours	⟷	3:30 pm
1600 hours	⟷	4:00 pm
2100 hours	⟷	9:00 pm
2352 hours	⟷	11:52 pm

An easy method to remember: To convert from regular time to the 24-hour clock, simply add 12 to the hour (starting at 1:00 pm):

$$3:30 \text{ pm} \rightarrow (\text{think } 3 + 12 = 15) \rightarrow 1530 \text{ hours}$$
$$11:52 \text{ pm} \rightarrow (\text{think } 11 + 12 = 23) \rightarrow 2352 \text{ hours}$$

To convert from the 24-hour clock to regular time, subtract 12 from the hour:

$$2100 \text{ hours} \rightarrow (\text{think } 21 - 12 = 9) \rightarrow 9:00 \text{ pm}$$
$$1745 \text{ hours} \rightarrow (\text{think } 17 - 12 = 5) \rightarrow 5:45 \text{ pm}$$

Figure 3-9 Introduction to the 24-hour clock.

- *Dosage.* This includes the amount of the drug and the strength of the preparation (e.g., two 100-mg tablets as opposed to 50-mg tablets or 250-mg tablets). It also includes when and how often the drug is to be taken (e.g., with meals or twice a day). The dosage portion of the order should tell whether it is a standing order or a self-terminating order (see pp. 56–57). You will learn more about dosages in Chapter 4.

- *Route of administration.* This is important because some medicines can be given by several different routes. If no special route is ordered, you can usually assume that the medication is to be taken orally. If in doubt, ask your supervisor.

- *Physician's signature.* Without the signature of the physician, the medication order is not legal. When a nurse or other staff member must take an order by phone, the nurse signs the order, and the physician co-signs it the next time he or she visits the health facility. When a physician prescribes drugs for clinic outpatients or private patients, the medication order will also include:

- *Number of refills.* Some drugs, especially Schedule II drugs, may not be refilled without another prescription. For other drugs, the order may show a certain number of refills. Figure 3-8 shows the number of refills, following the Latin word *repetatur,* meaning "repeat."

- *Labeling instructions.* These tell the pharmacist what instructions to put on the bottle for the patient—for example, "Take one tablet daily at bedtime." Labeling instructions are preceded by the abbreviation "sig," meaning "signature" or "write on label."

- *Quantity.* Outpatient prescriptions must specify the quantity of the drug to be dispensed to patient.

- *Physician's DEA number.* This is a registration number from the DEA. It is required on all prescriptions for controlled substances.

STANDING OR SELF-TERMINATING?

There are two basic types of medication orders: standing and self-terminating. A **standing order** is one that remains in force for an indefinite period of time. The medication may continue to be given until one of three things happens: (1) the physician writes a new order that cancels the old standing order; (2) the patient's condition improves to some specified level (e.g., the order may state, "Give aspirin, 650 mg, every 4 hours until temperature drops below 101° F"); or (3) the order is canceled automatically by agency policy. Some health facilities have a policy of canceling all standing orders after a certain amount of time, such as 4 weeks. This is done to make sure that physicians regularly recheck the medication needs of their patients.

Standing orders sometimes include the instruction to give as necessary, abbreviated PRN (for the latin phrase *pro re nata,* meaning "according to circumstances," also written p.r.n., prn, or P.R.N.). A PRN order gives the nurse or other health worker some choice in deciding when and how often to give the medication.

The other type of medication order is the **self-terminating order,** also known as the **automatic stop order (ASO).** This type of order puts a limit on how long the medication may be given. It states either a set amount of time or a set number of doses, for example:

Ergotrate maleate 0.2 mg, 1 tab. q8h × 48 h
or
Demerol 100 mg IM q4h × 12h and then PRN

Another example of a self-terminating order is a **stat order** (from the Latin term *statim*). This is an order to be carried out immediately and only once.

In some hospitals, orders are automatically terminated after surgery or when moving a patient to another clinic (e.g., from intensive care into a regular ward). The patient's medications must be reviewed at this time and new orders written.

In addition, certain types of drugs carry automatic stop orders as a matter of hospital policy. These drugs are antibiotics, narcotics, corticosteroids, anticoagulants, and barbiturates.

QUESTIONING A MEDICATION ORDER

There will be times when you have questions about a medication order. Perhaps you cannot read the doctor's handwriting. The prescribed dosage may seem unusually high or not quite right for your patient. You may find that a certain drug is not tolerated well by a patient. Or the patient may have trouble taking the drug by the prescribed route. When these questions come up, it is your right and your duty to check the order with the doctor or supervisor. In no case should you give a medication unless the orders are clearly written or stated.

What if your supervisor and the physician have explained the medication order to you, and still you are not satisfied that the medication is safe for the patient? You have the right to refuse to give any medication that you feel would endanger the patient. But ask your questions first. In most cases, the reasons behind the medication order will become clear.

TABLE 3-3: Time Abbreviations

ABBREVIATION (LATIN[a])	MEANING	TIMES GIVEN[b]
a.c. (ante cibum)	before meals	1/2 hour before a meal
ad lib. (ad libitum)	at pleasure	given freely, as much as is wanted
AM, A, a.m. (ante meridiem)	before noon	morning
BID, b.i.d. (bis in die)	twice a day	10 a.m. and 4 p.m.
h. (hora)	hourly	on each hour
h.s. (hora somni)	hour of sleep	at bedtime
n., noc. (nocte)	night	in the night
p.c. (post cibum)	after meals	1/2 hour after a meal
PM, P, p.m. (post meridiem)	after noon	afternoon
PRN, p.r.n. (pro re nata)	according to circumstances; occasionally, as necessary	repeat whenever
q.d., QD (quaque die)	every day	10 a.m. or as ordered
q.h., qq.h., (quaque hora)	every hour	on each hour
q2h, q.2h.	every 2 hours	6 a.m. and on even hours
q3h, q.3h.	every 3 hours	6, 9, 12, 3, day and night
q4h, q.4h.	every 4 hours	8, 12, 4, day and night
QID, q.i.d. (quater in die)	4 times a day	8 a.m., 12 noon, 4 p.m., 8 p.m.
q.o.d.		10 a.m. or as ordered
stat (statim)		given once as ordered
TID, t.i.d. (ter in die)		usually given with meals

[a] The Latin words are included only to show where the abbreviations come from. You do not need to memorize them.

[b] Medication schedules vary with different health facilities, so the specific times may vary according to where you work.

TABLE 3-4: Medical Abbreviations

ABBREVIATION (LATIN)	MEANING
a *(ante)*	before
AD *(aura dexter)*	right ear
AS *(aura sinister)*	left ear
AU *(aura uterque)*	both ears
c̄. *(cum)*	with
°C	degrees Celsius (Centigrade)
dil. *(dilue)*	dilute
°F	degrees Fahrenheit
♀	female
M *(misce)*	mix
♂	male
n.p.o. *(nil per os)*	nothing by mouth
non rep. *(non repetatur)*	do not repeat
OD *(oculus dexter)*	right eye
ophth., op. *(ophthalmicus)*	ophthalmic
OS *(oculus sinister)*	left eye
OU *(oculus uterque)*	both eyes
per *(per)*	by
p *(post)*	after
pH	acid/base balance (on a scale of 0 to 14)
PO, p.o. *(per os)*	by mouth
q., qq. *(quaque)*	every
q.s. *(quatum satis)*	a sufficient amount; as much as necessary
®	registered product name
Rx *(recipe)*	take
s̄. *(sine)*	without
sig. *(signa)*	directions
S̄S̄	one-half

a   Latin words are for reference only. You do not need to memorize them.

It is also important to know your agency's policies concerning which staff members are allowed to carry out which procedures. You should not be asked to carry out any procedure that is against agency policy.

STANDARD MEDICAL ABBREVIATIONS

Abbreviations are a shorthand form used to write medication orders. They are a quick, convenient way to summarize instructions on what drug to give and how to give it. Certain standard abbreviations are familiar to most people in the medical field. Tables 3-3 and 3-4 show some abbreviations commonly used in the medical profession.

It is traditional for doctors to write medication orders in Latin, the language of medicine. Most of the standard abbreviations they use on medication orders are shortened versions of Latin words. At times, this leads to confusion for those who have to interpret the instructions. Many people in the medical profession are now urging doctors to write out medication orders in plain English, without abbreviations. Nevertheless, the Latin abbreviations are still used by many physicians, as well as nurses and other health care workers.

It is important for you to memorize standard medical abbreviations to enable you to read and understand any medication order that you are expected to carry out. At some time, you may also have to translate a prescription into simple language for a patient's family.

◆ **NOTE** ◆ ◆ ◆ ◆ ◆ ◆ ◆ ◆ ◆ ◆ ◆ ◆ ◆ ◆ ◆ ◆ ◆ ◆

You may find abbreviations capitalized on some orders and not capitalized on others. You may also find differences in punctuation. The use of capital letters and periods is inconsistent in the profession. Check to see if your agency has its own list of approved abbreviations, and follow that list.

CHAPTER 3 REVIEW

Using Medical Terminology

Define each of the terms listed below.

1. Active ingredient _____

_____

2. Counterirritant _____

_____

3. Irrigation _____

_____

4. Inhalation _____

_____

5. Instillation _____

_____

6. Outpatient _____

_____

7. Physician's order sheet _____

_____

8. Self-terminating order _____

_____

9. Standing order _____

_____

10. Stat order _____

_____

Acquiring Knowledge of Medications

Match the forms of medication to their descriptions.

_____ 11. Heavy sugar and water solution with flavoring

_____ 12. Alcohol mixed with a volatile oil

_____ 13. 10–20% drug solution in alcohol and/or water

_____ 14. Highly concentrated alcohol solution

_____ 15. 10–20% drug solution in alcohol and water *plus* sweeteners and aromatics

_____ 16. Oils and fats suspended in water

_____ 17. Mixture of heavy particles with water; looks like milk

_____ 18. Thick mixture of fine particles with water

_____ 19. A soothing or counterirritant preparation for external use, designed to be rubbed in

_____ 20. A soothing or counterirritant preparation for external use, designed to be patted on

_____ 21. A topical or ophthalmic preparation in a base of lanolin or petrolatuma.

a. ointment
b. gel
c. emulsion
d. fluidextract
e. spirit
f. syrup
g. tincture
h. elixir
i. magma
j. liniment
k. lotion

Match the route to the proper abbreviation.

_____ 22. Under the tongue

_____ 23. Under the skin

_____ 24. Into the skin

_____ 25. Into the muscle

_____ 26. Into the vein

_____ 27. By mouth

_____ 28. Inside the cheek

a. buc
b. PO
c. ID
d. IV
e. subl
f. subcu
g. IM

Match the appropriate abbreviation to each phrase.

_____ 29. Eye medication orders

_____ 30. Medications given as necessary

_____ 31. Administration times

_____ 32. Before or after meals

_____ 33. Medications given once a day

_____ 34. Immediate, one-time order

_____ 35. Nothing by mouth

_____ 36. Chemical symbols

a. stat
b. BID, QID, q4h, h.s., a.m.
c. a.c., p.c.
d. HCl, NaCl, H_2O
e. ad lib., PRN
f. q.d.
g. NPO
h. OD, OS, OU, ophth.

Write the term that the abbreviation stands for.

37. Ext. _____

38. Syr. _____

39. Tinc. _____

40. Supp. _____

41. Sp. _____

42. Fld. ext. _____

43. Cap. _____

44. Elix. _____

45. Tab. _____

46. Soln. _____

47. Susp. _____

Describe the following solid forms.

48. Troche _____

_____

_____

49. Suppository _____

_____

50. Delayed-release capsule _____

_____

51. Scored tablet _____

_____

Fill in the blanks with the word or phrase that best completes each statement.

52. Because of their high drug concentrations, spirits, tinctures, and fluidextracts must be measured with a

_____

53. To prevent alcohol solutions from separating, store them in _____

54. Bottles containing tinctures, fluidextracts, elixirs, and spirits are kept tightly closed so that the

_____ cannot evaporate.

55. All suspensions must be _____ before use.

56. When a drug dissolves in water or alcohol, the resulting solution is called a(n) _____

57. When a drug does not dissolve in liquid, the preparation is called a(n) _____

58. _____ coated capsules and tablets prevent stomach irritation by dissolving only when they reach the intestine.

59. Highly concentrated powders of drugs are known as dry _____

60. Suppositories may be inserted into the _____, the _____, or the

_____ .

61. A diagnosed alcoholic should not be given any _____ solutions.

62. Delayed-release capsules are also called _____ .

63. Oral medicines are made to taste good to help _____ as well as _____ take them.

64. Elixirs of phenobarbital or *Benadryl* have _____ to make them _____ to help the elderly take them.

65. In sublingual and buccal administrations, no _____ is permitted until the medication is dissolved.

66. Applying local medications to the skin or the mucous membranes is known as the _____ route.

67. Injecting medications into the body with a needle and syringe is known as the _____ route.

68. Parenteral medications and equipment must be _____; otherwise, there is danger of infection.

Convert from the 24-hour clock to the regular clock and vice versa.

	Regular Clock	24-Hour Clock
69.	7:00 a.m.	_____
70.	_____	1100 hours
71.	_____	1330 hours
72.	2:00 p.m.	_____
73.	_____	2000 hours

Applying Knowledge on the Job

Answer the questions below in the spaces provided.

74. What should you do if you have a question about a medication order? _____
_____

75. What two new members of the health team, as well as doctors, are allowed to prescribe medications in some states? _____
_____

76. What is the important rule to remember when administering delayed-release tablets and capsules? Why is this rule important? _____
_____
_____

77. List six items of information that must be included on any written medication order.
_____
_____
_____
_____
_____
_____
_____

Translate the doctor's orders. Use your knowledge of medical abbreviations to give the meanings of the following orders.

78. Darvon caps 65 mg q4h PRN for pain _____

_____

_____

79. Phenobarbital elix. 1 tsp (20 mg) h.s. _____

_____

_____

80. Keflex 250 mg caps q6h PO _____

_____

_____

81. Lotrimin 1% cream bid × 2 weeks. _____

_____

_____

82. Bacitracin ophth. oint. OD TID for conjunctivitis _____

_____

83. Propantheline bromide tabs. 15 mg a.c. _____

_____

84. Heparin 5000 units IV stat _____

_____

85. Acetaminophen 120 mg r supp. QID _____

_____

→ ANSWERS TO CHAPTER 3 REVIEW ←

Using Medical Terminology

1. The ingredient in a product that produces the therapeutic effect.

2. A drug that irritates tissues so as to relieve some other problem.

3. Rinsing a body cavity with water or other solutions.

4. Administering drugs by way of droplets or mist that is breathed in.

5. Placing drops of liquid into the eyes, ears, nose, or some other body cavity.

6. Patient who is not hospitalized or institutionalized; a walk-in (or ambulatory) patient.

7. A form for writing out medication orders, located in the patient's chart.

8. Drug order that stops at a certain time or after a certain number of doses; also called automatic stop order.

9. Drug order that is to be continued until further notice.

10. Drug order carried out immediately and only once.

Acquiring Knowledge of Medications

11. f	12. e	13. g	14. d
15. h	16. c	17. i	18. b
19. j	20. k	21. a	22. e
23. f	24. c	25. g	26. d
27. b	28. a	29. h	30. e
31. b	32. c	33. f	34. a
35. g	36. d		

37. Extract

38. Syrup

39. Tincture

40. Spirit

41. Suppository

42. Fluidextract

43. Capsule

44. Elixir

45. Tablet

46. Solution

47. Suspension

48. Pleasant-tasting tablet made to dissolve in the mouth for a local effect

49. Drug held in a firm substance that melts at body temperature; designed for insertion in the vagina, rectum, or urethra

50. Capsule containing multiple doses of medicine that are released gradually for a sustained effect

51. Tablet with a groove down the middle for easy dividing

52. medicine dropper or medicine glass

53. a dark place

54. alcohol

55. shaken

56. solution

57. suspension

58. Enteric

59. extracts

60. rectum, vagina, urethra

61. alcohol

62. sustained-release or timed-release

63. old as well as young

64. added ingredients, tasting better

65. food or drink

66. topical

67. parenteral

68. sterile

69. 0700 hours

70. 11:00 a.m.

71. 1:30 p.m.

72. 1400 hours

73. 8:00 p.m.

Applying Knowledge on the Job

74. If you question a medication order, ask the doctor or the nurse in charge to explain the reasons for the order.

75. Physician's assistants and nurse practitioners.

76. Do not dissolve the contents of a delayed-release capsule in food or drink. In doing so, you might overdose the patient.

77. Patient's full name, date of the order, drug name, dosage (frequency, amount, strength), route of administration, signature of physician.

78. *Darvon* capsules, 65 mg every 4 hours as necessary for pain.

79. Phenobarbital elixir, 1 teaspoon (20 mg) at bedtime.

80. *Keflex* 250-mg capsules every 6 hours orally.

81. *Lotrimin* 1% cream twice a day for 2 weeks.

82. *Bacitracin* ophthalmic ointment in the right eye three times a day for conjunctivitis.

83. Propantheline bromide tablets, 15 mg before meals.

84. Heparin 5000 units intravenously immediately.

85. Acetaminophen 120-mg rectal suppository four times a day.

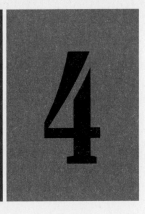

CHAPTER

4

Measurement and Dosage Calculation

◆◆   In this chapter you will learn about three systems used in measuring doses of medication. You will learn how to solve simple dosage problems and how to convert doses from one system of measurement to another. A review of fractions is included to help you brush up on your math skills.

COMPETENCIES

After studying this chapter, you should be able to

- write and define the abbreviations for units of measurement in the metric, apothecaries', and household systems.
- state the most common equivalents among apothecaries', metric, and household measures and use a conversion table to find less common equivalents.
- convert grams to milligrams and vice versa.
- convert milliliters to teaspoons and vice versa.
- calculate the number of tablets or capsules to give when the available dose differs from the ordered dose.
- calculate doses using a procedure for converting between different units of measurement.
- tell the difference between a child and an adult in dose calculation.
- calculate drops per minute for IV therapy.

VOCABULARY

Arabic numerals: 1, 2, 3, 4, and so on

centimeter: one-hundredth of a meter

convert: to change from one unit of measurement to another

dosage range: the different amounts of a drug that will produce therapeutic effects but not serious side effects or toxicity

fraction: a mathematical way of talking about an amount that is part of a whole or a ratio between two numbers

grain: basic unit of weight in the apothecaries' system

gram: basic unit of weight in the metric system

kilometer: 1000 meters

liter: basic unit of volume in the metric system

meter: basic unit of length in the metric system

metric system: a decimal system of measurement based on the meter and kilogram

milliliter: one-thousandth of a liter (same as cubic centimeter)

millimeter: one-thousandth of a meter

minim: basic unit of volume in the apothecaries' system

Roman numerals: I, II, III, IV, V, or i, ii, iii, iv, v, and so forth

unit: (1) basic quantity in a measurement system; (2) a way of telling the strength of hard-to-measure drugs such as antibiotics (e.g., 100,000 units of penicillin)

SYSTEMS OF MEASUREMENT

Measurement has always been an important part of prescribing and administering medications. This is so because different amounts of a drug give different effects. Some drugs are deadly poisons, but when given in tiny amounts, they can help relieve disorders. Other drugs are useless for therapy unless given in large amounts.

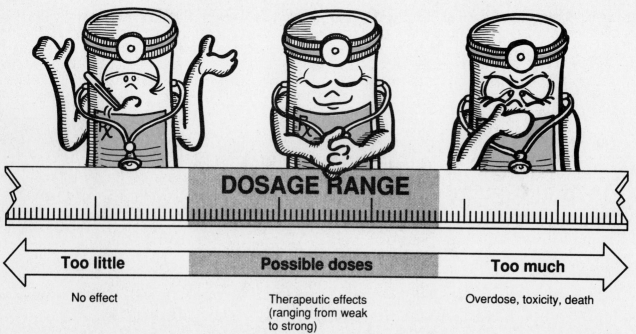

Figure 4-1 The physician chooses a certain dose within the dosage range according to the needs of the individual patient.

Most drugs have a certain **dosage range,** that is, different amounts that can produce therapeutic effects (Figure 4-1). Doctors prescribe an amount within the dosage range, depending on how strong an effect is needed and on the patient's age and physical condition. Doses below the dosage range will not produce the desired therapeutic effect. Doses above the dosage range can be harmful to the body and may be fatal.

To get the drug effects they want, physicians and pharmacists try to make dosages exact by measuring drugs carefully. However, they have not always used the same units of measurement. There are different measurement systems, each having its own units of weight and volume.

Today, three different systems of measurement are commonly used in the medical field. You should be familiar with the units of weight and volume found in each system. Dosages on a medication order may be expressed in units ranging from milliliters (or cubic centimeters) to drops, teaspoons, drams, or minims. You need to know what each of these quantities means so that you can measure out the doses properly. In addition, you may be asked to convert (change) from one unit or system to another in the course of your daily routine. You need to know how to use conversion tables to convert from milligrams to grams, from milliliters to teaspoons, from grains to milligrams, and so forth.

The three systems of measurement used in ordering medications are the apothecaries' system, the metric system, and the household system.

Apothecaries' System

The apothecaries' system of measurement is very old. It was brought to the United States from England during the eighteenth century. Colonial pharmacists (apothecaries) used it when compounding and measuring their medicinal preparations. The system is gradually being phased out in favor of the easier-to-use metric system.

The basic unit of weight in the apothecaries' system is the **grain** (gr). It was originally supposed to be the weight of one grain of wheat. The basic unit of volume is the **minim** (min). A minim is the space taken up by a quantity of water that weighs the same as a grain of wheat.

Table 4-1 lists all of the units of weight and volume in the apothecaries' system. Note especially the abbreviations for these units. You need to be able to recognize them on a medication order and write them on a medication chart.

In the apothecaries' system, dosage quantities are written out in lowercase **Roman numerals** (see Table 4-2). By convention the Roman numerals are written with a bar over them after the unit of measurement; for example, ℥ ī̄ī means 2 drams.

If the quantity of units is higher than 15, **Arabic** numerals can be used (15, 16, 17, etc.). Arabic numerals are usually written before the unit of measurement

---

TABLE 4-1: The Apothecaries' System

WEIGHT (DRY)	VOLUME (LIQUID)
grain (gr)	minim (min, ♍)
dram (dr or ℥)	fluidram (fl dr, ℥ or f ℥)
ounce (oz or ℥)	fluidounce (fl oz, ℥ or f ℥)
pound	pint (pt)
ton	quart (qt)

EQUIVALENTS
A minim of liquid weighs 1 grain
60 grains or 60 minims = 1 dram or fluidram
8 drams or fluidrams = 1 ounce or fluidounce

(e.g., 25 gr.), although many people prefer to write them after the unit to avoid confusing grains with grams in the metric system. Quantities less than 1 (e.g., (½, ¾) and mixed fractions (e.g., 2 ¾, 4 ½) are also usually written with Arabic numerals before the unit. The only exception is the quantity ½, for which the symbol $\overline{ss}$ is used with Roman numerals after the unit.

Here are some examples:

$$f \, \overline{\mathfrak{z}} \, v\overline{\imath\imath} = 7 \text{ fluidounces}$$

$$\overline{\mathfrak{z}} \, \overline{iv} = 4 \text{ drams}$$

$$gr \, \overline{iss} = 1 \text{ ½ grains}$$

$$5 \text{ ¼ } dr = 5 \text{ ¼ drams}$$

$$\text{⅟}_{150} \, gr \text{ (also gr ⅟}_{150}) = \text{⅟}_{150} \text{ grain}$$

$$15 \, gr \text{ (also gr 15)} = 15 \text{ grains}$$

$$30 \, min = 30 \text{ minims}$$

Metric System

The metric system is used throughout the world and is gradually becoming accepted in the United States, especially in medicine. It is a simple, logical system of measurement based on units of 10.

A unit of length, the **meter,** is the foundation of the metric system. It is actually one 10-millionth of the distance between the North Pole and the Equator. Metric volume is measured in fractions of a **liter** (L,l). Weight is measured in **grams** (g).

Prefixes added to the words *meter, gram,* and *liter* indicate smaller or larger units in the system (see Table 4-3). All units are a result of either multiplying or dividing by 10, 100, or 1000. The **centimeter,** for example, is 1/100th of a meter. A **millimeter** is 1/1000th of a meter. A **kilometer** is 1000 meters.

In the metric system, units of length, weight, and volume are related to each other in systematic ways. The unit of volume most often used in preparing medications is the **milliliter** (ml), which is one-thousandth of a liter. One milliliter is

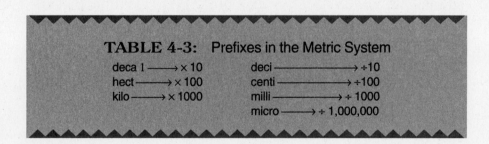

TABLE 4-3: Prefixes in the Metric System

deca 1 ⟶ × 10		deci ⟶ ÷10	
hect ⟶ × 100		centi ⟶ ÷100	
kilo ⟶ × 1000		milli ⟶ ÷ 1000	
		micro ⟶ ÷ 1,000,000	

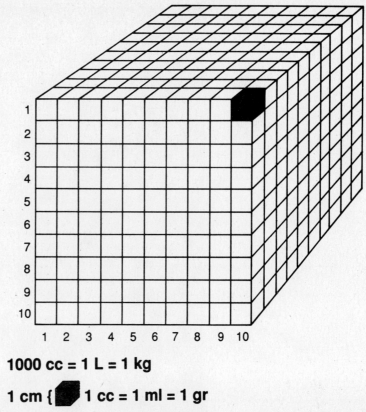

1000 cc = 1 L = 1 kg

1 cm { 1 cc = 1 ml = 1 gr

Figure 4-2 Relationships among units of length, volume, and weight in the metric system.

the liquid contents of a cube measuring 1 centimeter (cm) on a side, or 1 cubic centimeter (cc). One liter is the liquid contents of a cube measuring 10 cm on a side, or 1000 cc. One gram is equal to the weight of 1 ml (or cc) of water. One liter contains 1000 ml of water, so it weighs 1000 g (1 kilogram). These relationships are shown in Figure 4-2.

Metric doses are always written out in Arabic numerals. Fractions of metric doses are written as decimal fractions. For example, one-half gram is 0.5 g. In reading medication orders, pay special attention to where the decimal point is placed. The differences between 0.05 g, 0.5 g, and 5.0 g are huge when it comes to doses of medicine. A mistake could be dangerous.

Table 4-4 lists the basic units of volume and weight in the metric system and their equivalents. The bottom of the table shows how to change from milligrams to grams and vice versa. Note especially the instructions, because these are simple conversions you will probably make often on the job. The conversions are easy if you remember the hints shown in Table 4-4.

Household System

The household system of measurement is actually more complicated than the metric and apothecaries' systems. However, most of us have grown up using its basic units—feet, inches, miles, pints, quarts, pounds, and so on—so the household system is quite familiar to us.

For medical purposes, household measures are not as accurate as apothecaries' or metric measures. So why use them at all? The reason is that medicine orders sometimes have to be translated into terms that patients can understand and use on their own. Particularly in home care, patients need to be able to take medicines in doses that can be measured with utensils they have on hand (teaspoons, tablespoons, medicine droppers, etc.).

TABLE 4-4: The Metric System

WEIGHT
microgram (μg; mcg)
milligram (mg, mgm)
gram (g, Gm, gm)
kilogram (kg),

VOLUME
milliliter (ml)
cubic centimeter (cc, cm³)
liter (L, l)

EQUIVALENTS
One milliliter (1 ml) is the same as 1 cubic centimeter (1 cc), and for water, both weigh 1 gram
1000 milliliters = 1 liter = 1000 cubic centimeters
1000 micrograms = 1 milligram
1000 milligrams = 1 gram
1000 grams = 1 kilogram
100 milligrams = 0.1 gram
10 milligrams = 0.01 gram, etc.

SIMPLE CONVERSIONS

From grams to milligrams
g × 1000 = mg
Hint: Move decimal point three places to the right
0.25 g = 250 mg

From milligrams to grams
mg ÷ 1000 g
Hint: Move decimal point three places to the left
500 mg = .500 g = 0.5 g

The basic units of the household system are listed in Table 4-5. All household doses are written out in Arabic numerals.

TABLE 4-5: The Household System

WEIGHT (DRY)
ounce (oz)
pound (lb)
ton

VOLUME (LIQUID)
drop (gt): drops (gtt)
teaspoon (t, tsp)
tablespoon (T, tbsp)
teacup (6 oz)
cup (c) or glass (8 oz)
pint (pt)
quart (qt)
gallon (gal)

EQUIVALENTS
16 ounces = 1 pound
3 teaspoons = 1 tablespoon = 1/2 ounce
16 tablespoons = 1 cup = 8 fluidounces
2 cups = 1 pint
2 pints = 1 quart
4 quarts = 1 gallon

Drugs That Are Hard to Measure

Certain antibiotics and hormones from animal sources are impossible to weigh and measure in ordinary ways. Their strength is judged by the quantity shown to cause certain effects in laboratory animals and human volunteers—the bioassay technique. Rather than being dispensed in grams or grains, these drugs are dispensed in solutions labeled with a certain number of **units** (U) per cubic centimeter or milliliter. Examples of these drugs are penicillin and insulin.

CONVERTING BETWEEN MEASUREMENT SYSTEMS

From time to time you will find it necessary to change, or convert, from one system of measurement to another. A physician will order medicine in grains, but the hospital pharmacy may send up the medication in grams. Or perhaps an order written for milliliters will have to be converted into teaspoons for a patient who will be taking the medicine at home. These types of conversions are usually performed by the pharmacist or the nurse in charge. But other health workers should also know how to make simple conversions by referring to a conversion table. Table 4-6 shows the equivalents between measures in the apothecaries', metric, and household systems. As you can see, the equivalents are not exact but approximate. A 10% error usually occurs in making conversions.

TABLE 4-6: Commonly Used Measurement System Equivalents[a]

APOTHECARIES'	METRIC	HOUSEHOLD
Liquid volume		
1 minim (♍ or min)	0.06 ml (or cc)	1 drop
15 minims	1 ml	15 drops (gtt)[b]
1 fluidram (f ℨ)	4-5 ml	1 teaspoon (60 gtt)
4 fluidrams	15 ml	1 tablespoon
1 fluidounce (f ℥)	30 ml	2 tablespoons (1 oz)
	180 ml	1 teacup (6 oz)
	240 ml	1 cup or glass (8 oz)
	500 ml	1 pint (16 oz)
	750 ml	1.5 pints (24 oz)
	1000 ml (1 L)	1 quart (32 oz)
Dry weight		
1/60 gr	1 mg	
1 gr	60 mg	
71/2 gr	500 mg (0.5 g)	
15 gr	1000 mg (1 g)	
60 gr (1 dram)	4 g	
1 oz	30 g	1 oz
	500 g	1.1 lb
	1000 g (1 kg)	2.2 lb

a Equivalents are approximate. For example, some institutions set 1 grain equal to 64 or 65 mg for grain/milligram conversions.

b This figure varies. The number of drops per milliliter depends on the substance being measured.

You can make most of the conversions you need if you know these basic equivalents:

$$1 \text{ mg} = 1/60 \text{ gr}$$
$$60 \text{ mg} = 1 \text{ gr}$$
$$1 \text{ g} = 15 \text{ gr}$$

If you can remember these, it is easy to work out other equivalents (Table 4-7).

A close look at Figure 4-3 should also be helpful. It shows the relative sizes of containers you might use to measure out doses in the various systems.

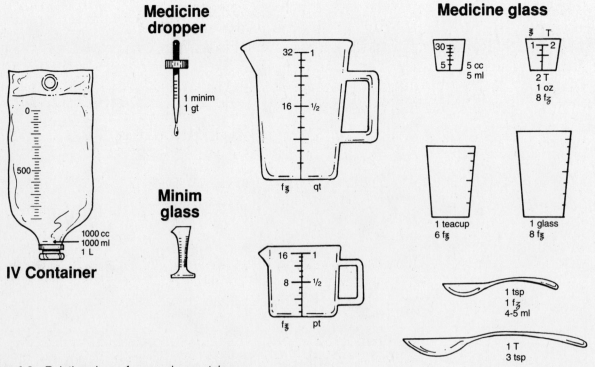

Figure 4-3 Relative sizes of measuring containers.

DOSAGE CALCULATION ◆◆

The job of calculating dosages is much easier today than in the past. Now in some health facilities pharmacists do all of the calculating. They prepare drugs in unit packages that contain the correct amount of a drug for a single dose. In your facility, however, you may have to make simple dosage calculations as part of your daily routine. You will need to know how to do this correctly and confidently. In medication administration there is no room for error!

In this section, you will learn two simple procedures that can be used to calculate almost any type of dosage problem. The only math you need to know is how to multiply and divide using whole numbers and fractions. Use paper and pencil to do your calculations, and check them carefully for errors. Some of the calculations are easy to do in your head. But practice with paper and pencil until you have mastered the techniques presented.

A brief review of fractions is included in this chapter. If your arithmetic skills are weak, you will need some extra practice. There are many books available in the library or bookstore to help you brush up on your basic skills.

Calculating the Number of Tablets, Capsules, or Milliliters

A type of calculation you will probably encounter is shown below.

Problem 1. The doctor orders 200 mg of a drug to be given three times a day. The pharmacy sends up a bottle of 50-mg capsules. You have to decide how many capsules to give for each dose.

A simple formula can be used to help you figure this out. The formula is:

Desired dose (what you WANT)	÷	Available dose per tablet, capsule, ml (what you HAVE)	=	Number of tablets, capsules, ml

or

$$\frac{\text{WANT}}{\text{HAVE}} = \text{Number of tablets or capsules, ml}$$

What this formula does is help you set up a fraction that you can simplify using the rules for fractions. Applying the formula to Problem 1, you get:

Dose ordered (WANT): 200 mg
Available packaging (HAVE): 50-mg caps

$$\frac{\text{WANT}}{\text{HAVE}} = \frac{200 \text{ mg}}{50 \text{ mg}} = \frac{\overset{4}{\cancel{200 \text{ mg}}}}{\underset{1}{\cancel{50 \text{ mg}}}} = 4 \text{ capsules}$$

Note that the units, mg, is also crossed out above and below the divider line when simplifying. The correct dose, then, would be four capsules three times a day.

Problem 2. The doctor orders 350 mg to be given once a day. All you have on hand are 100-mg tablets. How many tablets should you give? (If the drug ordered is a liquid, ml's or cc's can be used in place of tablets or capsules.)

$$\frac{\text{WANT}}{\text{HAVE}} = \frac{350 \text{ mg}}{100 \text{ mg}} = \frac{\overset{3.5}{\cancel{350 \text{ mg}}}}{\underset{1}{\cancel{100 \text{ mg}}}} = 3\ 1/2 \text{ tablets}$$

Note that your answer includes a fraction of a tablet. You may administer a half or a quarter of a tablet if the tablet is scored so that it breaks easily. If it is anything other than a scored tablet, ask the nurse in charge what to do. Dividing an unscored tablet is risky, and of course, you should not attempt to divide capsules or specially coated tablets.

Problem 3. Now try a problem involving another unit of measurement. You are to give 20 gr of aspirin to an arthritis patient. The aspirin tablets you have are 5 gr each. How many tablets do you give?

$$\frac{\text{WANT}}{\text{HAVE}} = \frac{\overset{4}{\cancel{20 \text{ gr}}}}{\underset{1}{\cancel{5 \text{ gr}}}} = 4 \text{ tablets}$$

Note that both WANT and HAVE must be in the same unit of measurement (e.g., both milligrams or grains, etc.). This formula does not apply to a problem like this:

$$\frac{100 \text{ mg}}{5 \text{ gr}}$$

Problem 4. What if the dosage ordered is a fractional dosage? For example, let's say that the doctor orders 1/2 gr and your tablets are 1/4 gr. Setting up the WANT/HAVE formula, you get:

$$(\text{Remember, this line means divided by}) \longrightarrow \frac{1/2 \text{ gr}}{1/4 \text{ gr}}$$

To work this out, use what you know about dividing fractions. You invert the bottom fraction and turn it into a multiplication problem:

$$\frac{1}{2} \div \frac{1}{4} = \frac{1}{\underset{1}{\cancel{2}}} \times \frac{\overset{2}{\cancel{4}}}{1} = 2 \text{ tablets}$$

Problem 5. The same procedure can be applied to situations where drugs are mixed into solutions. For example, the label on a bottle of elixir says that it contains 5 gr of medication per teaspoon. The doctor has ordered 15 gr of medication.

$$\frac{\text{WANT}}{\text{HAVE}} = \frac{\overset{3}{\cancel{15 \text{ gr}}}}{\underset{1}{\cancel{5 \text{ gr/tsp}}}} = 3 \text{ tsp}$$

Problem 6. It also works for units of penicillin mixed in sterile water for injection. A vial states that it contains 100,000 units of penicillin per cubic centimeter. You are to inject 300,000 units.

$$\frac{\text{WANT}}{\text{HAVE}} = \frac{\overset{3}{\cancel{300,000 \text{ units}}}}{\underset{1}{\cancel{100,000 \text{ units/cc}}}} = 3 \text{ cc}$$

Dosage Calculations with Conversions

Suppose that the doctor orders a dose in grams, but your capsules are labeled in milligrams. Perhaps the order is in grains and your tablets are labeled in milligrams. Or suppose that the order is in milliliters and you want to instruct the patient how much to take at home using a teaspoon.

Dosage calculations in which you need to convert from one system or unit of measurement to another cannot be handled by the simple WANT/HAVE formula. A more complex formula is needed, but it is easy to use and can be adapted to a variety of situations. The formula is:

$$\begin{array}{ccc}
\text{Dosage in ordered} & & \text{Conversion fraction} \\
\text{unit (KNOWN)} & \times & \text{(relation of} & = & \text{Dose in desired} \\
& & \text{UNKNOWN to} & & \text{unit (UNKNOWN)} \\
& & \text{KNOWN units)}
\end{array}$$

or

$$\text{KNOWN} \times \text{conversion fraction} = \text{UNKNOWN}$$

This formula is best explained in the context of some sample problems.

Problem 7. The doctor orders 0.5 g of ampicillin to be given four times a day. You want to know how many milligrams one dose would be. Your problem is:

$$0.5 \text{ g} = ? \text{ mg (KNOWN unit is 0.5 g; UNKNOWN unit is ? mg)}$$

To solve the problem, set up a calculation that will allow you to cancel the gram unit and give you the answer in milligrams.

$$\frac{0.5 \text{ g} \times ? \text{ mg}}{? \text{ g}} = \text{answer in milligrams}$$

You do this by means of a conversion fraction. This fraction differs according to the particular problem. It is designed to show the equivalence between the known and unknown units of measurement. The known type of unit should be in the denominator. For this problem, the conversion fraction is

$$\frac{? \text{ mg}}{? \text{ g}}$$

You must fill in the missing quantities.

First, you set the quantity of either unit to 1. Then you find out how many of the other units are contained in that quantity. In this case, let us set the quantity of grams at 1. One gram contains 1000 mg, so you fill in the fraction as follows:

$$\frac{1000 \text{ mg}}{1 \text{ g}}$$

Note that this fraction is equal to 1, because the numerator and the denominator both represent the same quantity, only in different units. Remember, the denominator must be in the same unit of measurement as the KNOWN dose.

Now you can solve the problem by first canceling the gram unit and multiplying:

$$0.5 \text{ g} \times \frac{1000 \text{ mg}}{1 \text{ g}} = 0.5 \times 1000 \text{ mg} = 500 \text{ mg}$$

Problem 8. Take another example, this one involving a conversion between household measures. You are to give a patient 6 tsp of milk of magnesia as necessary for constipation. How many tablespoons would that be? In other words, 6 tsp = ? T (KNOWN unit is 6 tsp, UNKNOWN is ? T).

Set up the calculation so that you can cancel out the teaspoons and get the answer in tablespoons:

$$6 \text{ tsp} \times \frac{? \text{ T}}{? \text{ tsp}} = \text{answer in tablespoons}$$

You know that 3 tsp = 1 T, so you can fill in the conversion fraction as 1 T/3 tsp. Proceed to solve as follows:

$$\cancel{6}^{2} \, \text{tsp} \times \frac{1 \, \text{T}}{\cancel{3} \, \text{tsp}} = 2 \, \text{T}$$

Problem 9. Next, try a problem that involves converting from one measurement system to another. The order is *Pro-Banthine* gr ss. You have tablets that are labeled in milligrams. Can you use the described procedure to find out how many milligrams equal 1/2 gr?

$$\frac{1}{2} \, \text{gr} \times \frac{? \, \text{mg}}{? \, \text{gr}} = \text{answer in mg}$$

From memory (or by looking at Table 4-7), you know that 1 gr = 60 mg, so:

$$\frac{1}{\cancel{2}} \, \cancel{\text{gr}} \times \frac{\cancel{60}^{30} \, \text{mg}}{1 \, \cancel{\text{gr}}} = 30 \, \text{mg}$$

Now, suppose that your tablets of *Pro-Banthine* are 15 mg each. How many 15-mg tablets would it take to make 30 mg? Some quick mental figuring tells you that you should give the patient two tablets. If in doubt, you can use the WANT/HAVE formula, now that you have already converted from grains to milligrams.

$$\frac{\text{WANT}}{\text{HAVE}} = \frac{\cancel{30}^{2} \, \text{mg}}{\cancel{15}_{1} \, \text{mg}} = 2 \, \text{tablets}$$

Children's Doses

As you learned in Chapter 2, children need smaller doses of medicine than adults. There are two ways to adjust dosages for children: by age and by weight. In both cases, you can use the basic KNOWN/UNKNOWN procedure you have just learned. But first, here is the way children and adults are defined for the purpose of calculating doses.

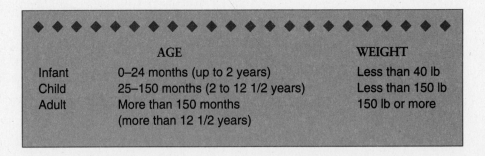

	AGE	WEIGHT
Infant	0–24 months (up to 2 years)	Less than 40 lb
Child	25–150 months (2 to 12 1/2 years)	Less than 150 lb
Adult	More than 150 months (more than 12 1/2 years)	150 lb or more

Adjusting Doses by Age. You should know how to check or verify pediatric doses. A 6-month-old infant is to be given tetracycline. The usual adult dose is 250 mg. You should set up the problem as follows:

$$\text{Patient's age (in months)} \times \frac{\text{Usual adult dose}}{\text{Adult age (in months)}}$$
$$= \text{Child's dose}$$

The adult age is always 150 months (12½ years) in this method of calculating. After filling in the proper numbers for your problem, you would get:

$$6 \text{ months} \times \frac{250 \text{ mg}}{150 \text{ months}} = \frac{1500 \text{ mg}}{150} = 10 \text{ mg}$$

The infant would therefore be given 10 mg of tetracycline.

Suppose that you were giving tetracycline to an 8-year-old child. Eight years is the same as 96 months (8 × 12 = 96), so your problem would look like this:

$$96 \text{ months} \times \frac{250 \text{ mg}}{150 \text{ months}} = \frac{24,000 \text{ mg}}{150} = 160 \text{ mg}$$

Adjusting Doses by Weight. You can figure out a child's dose by weight, just as you did by age. An adult is considered to weigh 150 lb in this formula:

$$\text{Patient's weight} \times \frac{\text{Usual adult dose}}{\text{Adult weight (always 150 lb)}} = \text{Child's dose}$$

A doctor orders *Dilantin* for a 30-lb child. The usual adult dose is 100 mg. Your calculation would look like this:

$$\overset{1}{30 \text{ lb}} \times \frac{100 \text{ mg}}{\underset{5}{150 \text{ lb}}} = \frac{100 \text{ mg}}{5} = 20 \text{ mg}$$

Parenteral Therapy

Another formula that is important to know is one used with intravenous (IV) therapy. You will work here with one simple formula, but books are available covering this subject in detail. This formula will allow you to calculate drops per minute for most physician's orders relating to this type of patient care. However, there are IV pumps and controllers that will figure rates.

Suppose that the doctor orders an infusion for a patient and specifies the amount of solution and the amount of time for it to be given. You will need to calculate the rate of flow or the number of drops per minute after you select the size of the IV tubing or drop factor. (The drop factor of the tubing for the adult is either 15 or 16 drops per 1 ml, and for the child it is 60 microdrops per 1 ml.) You will need the fraction 1 hour/60 minutes to complete the problem. The IV container will give you one of these drop factors.

Problem 10. The doctor orders 120 ml of 5% D/W to be given over a 6-hour period. The drop factor is 60 microdrops per 1 ml. How many microdrops would you administer in 1 minute?

$$120 \text{ ml in a 6-hour period} = \frac{120 \text{ ml}}{6 \text{ hour}}$$

Convert milliliters per hour to microdrops per minute:

$$\frac{120 \text{ ml}}{6 \text{ hour}} = \frac{? \text{ microdrops}}{? \text{ minutes}}$$

Write in one line as follows:

$$\frac{120 \text{ ml}}{6 \text{ hour}} \times \frac{60 \text{ microdrops}}{1 \text{ ml}} \times \frac{1 \text{ hour}}{60 \text{ minutes}}$$

Cancel the labels and the numbers that are equal:

$$\frac{\overset{20}{120 \text{ ml}}}{\underset{1}{6 \text{ hour}}} \times \frac{\overset{1}{60 \text{ microdrops}}}{1 \text{ ml}} \times \frac{1 \text{ hour}}{\underset{1}{60 \text{ minutes}}} = \frac{20 \text{ microdrops}}{1 \text{ minute}}$$

The order of 120 ml given over a 6-hour period would be administered at the rate of 20 microdrops per minute after you cancel and then multiply across terms.

Problem 11. How many drops per minute would you administer if the doctor ordered 1000 cc of 5% D/W in a 12-hour period?

$$1000 \text{ ml in a 12-hour period} = \frac{1000 \text{ cc}}{12 \text{ hour}}$$

Convert milliliters per hour to microdrops per minute:

$$\frac{1000 \text{ cc}}{12 \text{ hour}} = \frac{? \text{ gtt}}{? \text{ minutes}}$$

Write in one line as follows:

$$\frac{1000 \text{ cc}}{12 \text{ hour}} \times \frac{15 \text{ gtt}}{1 \text{ cc}} \times \frac{1 \text{ hour}}{60 \text{ minutes}}$$

Cancel the labels and the numbers that are equal:

$$\frac{\overset{250}{\cancel{1000} \text{ cc}}}{12 \text{ hour}} \times \frac{\overset{1}{\cancel{15} \text{ gtt}}}{1 \text{ cc}} \times \frac{1 \text{ hour}}{\underset{4}{\cancel{60}} \text{ minutes}} \times \frac{250}{12} = 20.8 \text{ or } \frac{21 \text{ gtt}}{1 \text{ minute}}$$

The order of 1000 cc given over a 12-hour period would be administered at the rate of 21 drops per minute.

When in Doubt

As a giver of medications, you share in the health care team's responsibility for making sure that the patient gets the correct dose. To meet this responsibility, you are learning all you can about dosage calculation and conversions between measurement systems. If you study hard and do the practice exercises until you have mastered them, you will be prepared to handle most routine dosage questions. However, you must also recognize your limitations. If you are the least bit confused about a conversion, or if you are unsure about a particular calculation, get help. Ask the physician, the nurse in charge, or the pharmacist to check your work. There should be no shame in asking for assistance in this area. After all, the main concern is the welfare of the patient. What could be more important than getting the dose right?

MATH REVIEW: FRACTIONS

DEFINITIONS
A **fraction** is a way of expressing an amount that is part of a whole:

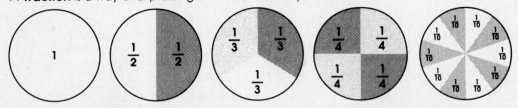

The more parts the whole is divided into, the smaller each part has to be:

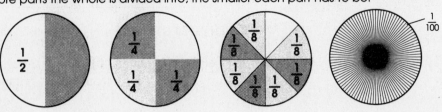

The whole can be a set of things, for example, nine dots or 100 mg:

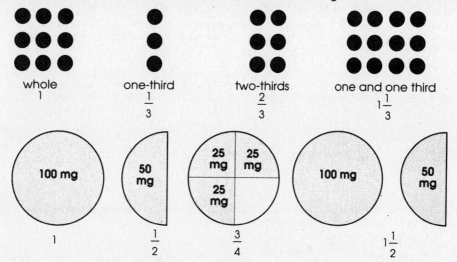

whole	one-third	two-thirds	one and one third
1	$\frac{1}{3}$	$\frac{2}{3}$	$1\frac{1}{3}$

A fractional amount of a whole is expressed like this:

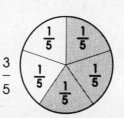

NUMERATOR: how many parts of the whole you are taking → $\frac{3}{5}$

DENOMINATOR: how many equal parts the whole is divided into →

A fraction is also a way of expressing a *relationship between two numbers* or quantities; for example $^3/_4$ means "3 divided by 4," which can also be expressed as:

$$3 \div 4 \quad \text{or} \quad 4\overline{)3} \quad \text{or} \quad 3 : 4 \quad \text{(ratio)}$$

A relationship like $\dfrac{350 \text{ mg}}{25 \text{ mg}}$ means the same as:

$$350 \text{ mg} \div 25 \text{ mg} \quad \text{or} \quad 25 \text{ mg}\overline{)350 \text{ mg}} \quad \text{or} \quad 350 \text{ mg} : 25 \text{ mg}$$

Simplifying fractions

To make calculations easier, fractions may be reduced to lowest terms:

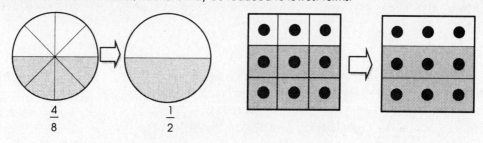

$$\frac{4}{8} = \frac{4 \div 4}{8 \div 4} = \frac{1}{2} \qquad \frac{6}{9} = \frac{6 \div 3}{9 \div 3} = \frac{2}{3}$$

To reduce a fraction to lowest terms, *divide* both the numerator and the denominator by the largest number that will go into both of them evenly. *(Note: If there is no number that goes into both the numerator and denominator evenly, you cannot reduce the fraction: it is already in lowest terms.)*

When you reduce a fraction, the amount stays the same, but the fraction is easier to work with.

Canceling is a short cut way of showing that you have divided the top and bottom of the fraction by the same number. Here is how it is shown in written work:

$\dfrac{3}{15}$ You wish to reduce 3/15 to the lowest terms, so you divide the top and bottom by the largest number that will go into both of them evenly, or 3.

$\dfrac{\cancel{3}^{1}}{\cancel{15}_{5}}$ Three goes into 3 once, so you cancel out the 3 and write 1.
Three goes into 15 five times, so you cancel out the 15 and write 5.

$\dfrac{1}{5}$ Thus, after reducing to lowest terms, the fraction is 1/5.

Units of measurement can be canceled too, as long as the same type of unit appears in both the numerator and the denominator.

$$\dfrac{18\,\cancel{mg}}{25\,\cancel{mg}} \quad or \quad \dfrac{3\,\cancel{gr}}{5\,\cancel{gr}} \quad but\ not \quad \dfrac{3\,gr}{50\,mg}$$

To simplify a "top heavy" fraction (or improper fraction) where the numerator is larger than the denominator, turn it into a mixed number (whole number and fraction) as follows:

Such top-heavy fractions are changed to mixed numbers *only* in giving the final answer to a problem. During calculations, mixed numbers are awkward to work with and must be changed to improper fractions.

Divide the numerator by the denominator. Express the remainder as a fraction with the same denominator.

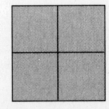 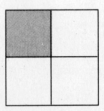

$$\dfrac{5}{4} = 1\dfrac{1}{4} \left(4\overline{)5}^{\,1\ rem\ 1} \right)$$

Multiplying Fractions

To multiply a fraction by another fraction, multiply *numerator x numerator* and *denominator x denominator* (x = times):

$$\dfrac{3}{10} \times \dfrac{1}{10} = \dfrac{3\times1}{10\times10} = \dfrac{3}{100}$$

$$\dfrac{5}{8} \times \dfrac{2}{3} = \dfrac{5\times2}{8\times3} = \dfrac{10}{24}$$

Remember to reduce the answer to lowest terms.

$$\dfrac{\cancel{10}^{5}}{\cancel{24}_{12}} = \dfrac{5}{12} \quad \text{(divided top and bottom by 2)}$$

To multiply a fraction by a whole number, multiply *whole number x numerator*.

(You may express the whole number as a fraction by giving it the denominator "1.") Then place the product over the denominator and simplify.

$$\dfrac{7}{9} \times 2 = \dfrac{7}{9} \times \dfrac{2}{1} = \dfrac{14}{9} = 1\dfrac{5}{9}$$

In multiplying fractions, you are allowed to cancel across the times sign as follows:

$$\frac{3}{\cancel{4}_{1}} \times \frac{\cancel{4}^{1}}{5} = \frac{3 \times 1}{1 \times 5} = \frac{3}{5}$$

$$\frac{\cancel{8}^{4}}{9} \times \frac{5}{\cancel{14}_{7}} = \frac{4 \times 5}{9 \times 7} = \frac{20}{63}$$

You divide the denominator of one fraction and the numerator of the opposite fraction by the same number. This makes your job easier because you work with smaller numbers.

In the same way, you may cancel identical units of measurment across the times sign. This is important for certain formulas in dosage calculation:

$$2 \cancel{tsp} \times \frac{5 \text{ ml}}{1 \cancel{tsp}} = 10 \text{ ml}$$

$$\cancel{7.5}^{.5} \cancel{gr} \times \frac{1 \text{ g}}{\cancel{15}_{1} \cancel{gr}} = 0.5 \text{ g}$$

Dividing fractions

Flip over (invert) the divisor and then *multiply* the two fractions:

$$\frac{1}{2} \div \overset{\text{invert}}{\underset{\downarrow}{\frac{2}{3}}} = \frac{1}{2} \times \frac{3}{2} = \frac{3}{4}$$

$$\frac{5}{8} \div \frac{5}{9} = \frac{\cancel{5}^{1}}{8} \times \frac{9}{\cancel{5}_{1}} = \frac{9}{8}$$

$$\frac{4}{5} \div 3 = \frac{4}{5} \times \frac{1}{3} = \frac{4}{15}$$

Decimal fractions

In working with metric measures, fractions are expressed as decimals. Here is how the decimal system works:

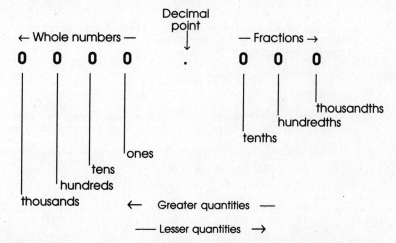

The placement of numbers in relation to the decimal point tells their values are multiples of 10.

Here are some examples of various whole numbers and fractions expressed as decimals:

$$1.0 \rightarrow 1\frac{0}{10} \rightarrow 1 \qquad\qquad 0.33 \rightarrow \frac{33}{100} \rightarrow \frac{1}{3}$$

$$0.75 \rightarrow \frac{75}{100} \rightarrow \frac{3}{4} \qquad\qquad 0.25 \rightarrow \frac{25}{100} \rightarrow \frac{1}{4}$$

$$0.66 \rightarrow \frac{66}{100} \rightarrow \frac{2}{3} \qquad\qquad 0.125 \rightarrow \frac{125}{1000} \rightarrow \frac{1}{8}$$

$$0.5 \rightarrow \frac{5}{10} \rightarrow \frac{1}{2}$$

As just shown, any decimal fraction can be expressed as a regular or common fraction. Note the position of the final digit relative to the decimal point;

$$0.48 \rightarrow \frac{48}{100} \rightarrow \frac{\cancel{48}^{12}}{\cancel{100}_{25}} \rightarrow \frac{12}{25}$$
hundredths

$$1.6 \rightarrow 1\frac{6}{10} \rightarrow 1\frac{\cancel{6}^{3}}{\cancel{10}_{5}} \rightarrow 1\frac{3}{5}$$
tenths

Any common fraction can be changed to a decimal fraction by dividing the numerator by the denominator:

$$\frac{1}{3} \rightarrow 3\overline{\big)\begin{array}{l}0.333,\text{etc.}\\1.00\end{array}} \rightarrow 0.33$$

$$\begin{array}{r}9\\\hline10\\9\\\hline1\end{array}$$

To multiply decimal fractions: $1.5 \times 0.35 = ?$

Set up your multiplication like a normal multiplication problem:

$$\begin{array}{r}1.5\\\times 0.35\\\hline75\\45\\\hline0.525\end{array}$$

To decide where the decimal point goes, look at the original problem and count the total number of places shown to the right of the decimal point, in this case 3.

$$1.5 \times 0.35 = 0.525$$
$$1 \qquad 23 \qquad 321$$

Then, starting from the last digit of the answer, count that many places to the left, and place the decimal right after that digit.

More examples:

$$100 \times 0.01 = 1.00$$
$$12 \qquad 21$$

$$3.25 \times 0.002 = 0.00650$$
$$12 \qquad 345 \qquad 54321$$

$$2.5 \times 1.4 = 3.50$$
$$1 \qquad 2 \qquad 21$$

Placing the decimal point correctly is *very* important. A misplaced decimal means a huge error in the dose.

Divide decimal fractions as follows: 30 ÷ 1.5 = ?

If there is a decimal fraction in the divisor, move it to the right past the rightmost digit, making the divisor a whole number. Count how many places you moved it. Then move the decimal in the dividend the same number of places to the right. The decimal should be placed directly above the point in the quotient (answer).

$$\begin{array}{r} 20. \quad\leftarrow \text{quotient} \\ \text{divisor} \rightarrow \ 1.5\,\overline{\smash{)}\,30.0}\quad\leftarrow \text{dividend} \end{array}$$

If there is no decimal fraction in the divisor, the quotient gets a decimal point directly above the one in the dividend.:

$$15\,\overline{\smash{)}\,30.0}\ \ \overset{2.0}{}$$

CHAPTER 4 REVIEW

Using Medical Terminology

Define each of the terms listed below.

1. Dosage range _____

_____

_____

2. Grain _____

_____

_____

3. Metric system _____

_____

_____

4. Minim _____

_____

_____

5. Unit _____

_____

_____

6. Liter _____

_____

_____

7. Meter _____

_____

8. Fraction _____

_____

9. Centimeter _____

_____

_____

10. Milliliter _____

_____

_____

Acquiring Knowledge of Medications

Write abbreviations for these units of measurement.

11. Minim _____   12. Tablespoon _____

13. Grain _____   14. Pound _____

15. Dram _____   16. Milligram _____

17. Fluidram _____   18. Milliliter _____

19. Ounce _____   20. Cubic centimeter _____

21. Drop _____   22. Liter _____

23. Pint _____   24. Gram _____

Practice decoding abbreviations. The following dosage orders are given using Roman numerals and abbreviations for the apothecaries' system of measurement. Write them out in full, using Arabic numerals.

25. $\frac{z}{3}$ iv _____   26. m ii _____

27. gr iss _____   28. f$\frac{z}{3}$ ix _____

Fill in the blanks. Refer to Tables 4-4, 4-6, and 4-7 if necessary.

29. A grain weighs the same as _____ minim(s) of liquid.

30. One minim is the same as _____ drop(s).

31. One milliliter is approximately equivalent to _____ drop(s).

32. Fifteen grains is about _____ gram(s).

33. One grain is about _____ milligram(s).

34. One gram is equal to _____ milligrams.

35. One milliliter is the same as _____ cubic centimeter(s).

36. One-half of a gram equals _____ milligram(s).

37. One liter (1000 cc) is about _____ quart(s).

Reduce these fractions to the lowest terms.

38. $^4/_8 =$ _____

39. $^{21}/_{28} =$ _____

40. $^3/_9 =$ _____

41. $^{250}/_{1000} =$ _____

42. $^{24}/_{32} =$ _____

43. $^{25}/_{45} =$ _____

Change these improper fractions to mixed numbers.

44. $^8/_3 =$ _____

45. $^{18}/_4 =$ _____

46. $^5/_2 =$ _____

47. $^{68}/_3 =$ _____

48. $^{17}/_{12} =$ _____

49. $^{350}/_{100} =$ _____

50. $^{55}/_{20} =$ _____

51. $^{27}/_5 =$ _____

Multiply these fractions and reduce them to the lowest terms.

52. $^3/_{10} \times ^1/_{10} =$ _____

53. $^5/_8 \times ^2/_3 =$ _____

54. $2 \times ^5/_8 =$ _____

55. $^5/_4 \times ^7/_6 =$ _____

56. $250 \text{ mg} \times 1 \text{ gr}/60 \text{ mg} =$ _____

57. $3 \text{ gr} \times 60 \text{ mg}/1 \text{ gr} =$ _____

Divide these fractions and reduce them to the lowest terms.

58. $^1/_2 \div ^2/_3 =$ _____

59. $^5/_8 \div ^5/_9 =$ _____

60. $^1/_{60} \div 3 =$ _____

61. $1 \div ^1/_{600} =$ _____

Write these fractions as decimals.

62. $^1/_2 =$ _____

63. $^1/_3 =$ _____

64. $^1/_4 =$ _____

65. $^2/_3 =$ _____

66. $^3/_4 =$ _____

67. $^6/_{10} =$ _____

68. $^{25}/_{100} =$ _____

69. $^{89}/_{100} =$ _____

70. $^{23}/_{1000} =$ _____

71. $3 \, ^3/_4 =$ _____

Change these decimals to fractions and reduce them to the lowest terms.

72. $0.75 =$ _____

73. $0.2 =$ _____

74. $1.5 =$ _____

75. $5.66 =$ _____

76. $0.005 =$ _____

77. $0.375 =$ _____

Multiply or divide these decimals as directed.

78. $1.5 \times 3 =$ _____

79. $1.5 \times 0.3 =$ _____

80. $1.5 \times 0.03 =$ _____

81. $2.75 \times 0.1 =$ _____

82. $7.5 \div 25 =$ _____

83. $7.5 \div 2.5 =$ _____

Convert from grams to milligrams or from milligrams to grams as directed.

84. $0.1 \text{ g} =$ _____ mg

85. $2.5 \text{ g} =$ _____ mg

86. $0.03 \text{ g} =$ _____ mg

87. $0.125 \text{ g} =$ _____ mg

88. $325 \text{ mg} =$ _____ g

89. $1200 \text{ mg} =$ _____ g

90. $3000 \text{ mg} =$ _____ g

91. $5 \text{ mg} =$ _____ g

Applying Knowledge on the Job

Solve the following problems.

92. 0.1 mg = _____ gr

93. 150 mg = _____ gr

94. 0.5 mg = _____ gr

95. _____ mg = 5 gr

96. _____ mg = ⅟₆₀ gr

97. 1 g = _____ gr

98. 4 mg = _____ gr

99. _____ g = 7 ½ gr

Use the WANT/HAVE formula to solve these dosage problems.

100. The doctor orders 250 mg of a drug. You have 100-mg scored tablets on hand. You will give the patient _____ tablets.

101. The medication order calls for a dose of 1¼ gr aspirin. Aspirin comes in scored tablets of 5 gr each. You will give the patient _____ tablet.

102. The physician orders 75 mg of a drug. You have capsules of 25 mg each. You give the patient _____ capsules.

103. An injectable antibiotic is packaged 100,000 units/cc. The doctor orders 400,000 units. A nurse will administer _____ to the patient parenterally.

104. A solution contains 25 mg of a drug per teaspoon. The doctor orders 50 mg. You give _____ tsp.

105. You have ½-gr tablets. You want to give ¼ gr. You administer _____ tablet(s).

106. The doctor's order is to give gr $\overline{xv}$. The medicine bottle shows that each 5-ml teaspoon contains 7½ gr. You give _____ tsp. (Hint: 7½ gr = ¹⁵∕₂ gr.)

Solve these dosage problems using Table 4-7 as a resource.

107. The doctor orders 600 mg. The dosage form on hand is gr $\overline{x}$ tablets. You give _____ tablet(s). (Hint: Find 600 mg = ? gr; then use the WANT/HAVE formula.)

108. You have ¼-gr tablets on hand, and the doctor has ordered 15 mg of the drug. You give _____ tablet(s).

109. The doctor ordered ¾ gr. The tablets on hand contain 30 mg each. You give _____ tablet(s). (Hint: Find ¾ gr = ? mg; then use the WANT/HAVE formula.)

110. An order is for 45 minims of a drug, but you do not have a measuring container marked in minims. You do have a container marked in milliliters. You administer _____ ml.

Translate each medication order and then answer the dosage questions.

111. An order reads "Hybephen f ℥ ī t.i.d. (PO) × 5 days."

   a. You do not have a glass container marked in fluidounces. What household measure could you use? _____

   _____

b. How many tablespoons are there in f℥ī? _____

c. How many fluidounces do you need for a 1-day supply of *Hybephen?* _____

d. How many fluidounces of *Hybephen* are needed in 5 days? _____

e. How many pints do you order from the pharmacy to have a 5-day supply of *Hybephen?* _____

112. An order reads "Fer-In-Sol 18 mg q.d.p.c." One teaspoon supplies 18 mg of iron. The pharmacy sends up an 8-oz bottle of Fer-In-Sol.

a. How many teaspoons are there in an 8-oz bottle (8 oz = ? tsp)? _____

b. About how many days will the bottle of *Fer-In-Sol* last? _____

Practice calculating dosages for children. The usual adult dose of Dilantin is 100 mg.

113. How much *Dilantin* would you give to a child 9 months old? _____

114. How much *Dilantin* would you give to a child who weighs 34 lb? _____

115. How much would you give to a 10-year-old? _____

116. How much would you give to a 16-year-old? _____

Practice calculating IV therapy doses.

117. How many drops per minute will you give if the order is 500 ml of 5% D/W in 5 hours? The drop factor is 15 gtt = 1 ml. _____

118. You are ordered to give the patient 500 cc of blood in 5 hours. Calculate the rate of flow. The drop factor is 20 gtt = 1 cc. (Remember, the tubing gives the drop factor, and for blood it can be 20 gtt = 1 cc instead of 15 or 16 gtt = 1 cc.) _____

119. The physician orders 1500 ml of 5% D/W in 24 hours. The drop factor is 15 gtt = 1 cc. How many drops per minute will you give? _____

120. Order: give 2000 cc of 5% D/W in 20 hours. Calculate the infusion rate if the drop factor is 15 gtt = 1 cc.
_____

➤ ANSWERS TO CHAPTER 4 REVIEW ◄

Using Medical Terminology

1. The different amounts of a drug that will produce therapeutic effects but not serious side effects or toxicity.

2. Basic unit of weight in the apothecaries' system.

3. A decimal system of measurement based on the meter and gram.

4. Basic unit of volume in the apothecaries' system.

5. Basic quantity in a measurement system or a way of telling the strength of hard-to-measure drugs such as antibiotics.

6. Basic unit of volume in the metric system.

7. Basic unit of length in the metric system.

8. A mathematical way of talking about an amount that is part of a whole or a ratio between two numbers.

9. One-hundredth of a meter.

10. One-thousandth of a liter, the same as a cubic centimeter.

Acquiring Knowledge of Medications

11. min, ♏ 12. T, tbsp
13. gr 14. lb
15. dr, ʒ 16. mg
17. fldr, f ʒ 18. ml
19. oz, ℥ 20. cc, cm^3
21. gtt 22. L, l
23. pt 24. g, gm
25. 4 drams 26. 2 minims
27. $1\frac{1}{2}$ grains 28. 9 fluidrams
29. 1 30. 1
31. 15 32. 1
33. 60 34. 1000
35. 1 36. 500
37. 1 38. $\frac{1}{2}$
39. $\frac{3}{4}$ 40. $\frac{1}{3}$
41. $\frac{1}{4}$ 42. $\frac{3}{4}$
43. $\frac{5}{9}$ 44. $2\frac{2}{3}$
45. $4\frac{1}{2}$ 46. $2\frac{1}{2}$
47. $22\frac{2}{3}$ 48. $1\frac{5}{12}$
49. $3\frac{1}{2}$ 50. $2\frac{3}{4}$
51. $5\frac{2}{5}$ 52. $\frac{3}{100}$
53. $\frac{5}{12}$ 54. $1\frac{1}{4}$
55. $1\frac{11}{24}$ 56. $4\frac{1}{6}$ gr
57. 180 mg 58. $\frac{3}{4}$
59. $1\frac{1}{8}$ 60. $\frac{1}{180}$
61. 600 62. 0.5
63. 0.333 64. 0.25
65. 0.667 66. 0.75
67. 0.6 68. 0.25
69. 0.89 70. 0.023
71. 3.75 72. $\frac{3}{4}$
73. $\frac{1}{5}$ 74. $1\frac{1}{2}$
75. $5\frac{2}{3}$ 76. $\frac{1}{200}$
77. $\frac{3}{8}$ 78. 4.5
79. 0.45 80. 0.045
81. 0.275 82. 0.3
83. 3 84. 100
85. 2500 86. 30
87. 125 88. 0.325
89. 1.2 90. 3
91. 0.005

Applying Knowledge on the Job

92. $\frac{1}{600}$ 93. $2\frac{1}{2}$
94. $\frac{1}{120}$ 95. 300
96. 1 97. 15
98. $\frac{1}{15}$ 99. 0.5
100. $2\frac{1}{2}$ ($\frac{250}{100} = 2\frac{1}{2}$)
101. $\frac{1}{4}$ $\left(\frac{\frac{5}{4}}{5} = \frac{5}{4} \times \frac{1}{5}\right)$ 102. 3 ($\frac{75}{25} = 3$)
103. 4 ($\frac{400{,}000}{100{,}000} = 4$) 104. 2 ($\frac{50}{25} = 2$)
105. $\frac{1}{2}$ $\left(\frac{\frac{1}{4}}{\frac{1}{2}} = \frac{1}{4} \times \frac{2}{1} = \frac{1}{2}\right)$
106. 2 $\left(\frac{15}{\frac{15}{2}} = 15 \times \frac{2}{15} = 2\right)$
107. 1 108. 1
109. $1\frac{1}{2}$ 110. 3

111. a. tablespoon
b. 2 T
c. f℥ $\overline{\text{iii}}$ (t.i.d. means three times a day, 3 × f℥ i = f℥ $\overline{\text{iii}}$)
d. f℥ $\overline{\text{xv}}$ (f℥ $\overline{\text{iii}}$ per day times 5 is f℥ $\overline{\text{xv}}$)
e. approx. 1 pt $\left(15 \cancel{\text{fl. oz.}} \times \frac{1 \text{ pt}}{16 \cancel{\text{fl. oz.}}} = \frac{15}{16} \text{ pt}\right)$

112. a. 48 tsp ((8 fl oz contains 16 T (see Table 4-6); to get teaspoons, multiply by 3 (or $16 \cancel{\text{T}} \times \frac{3 \text{ tsp}}{1 \cancel{\text{T}}} = 48$ tsp)))
b. 48 days (given q.d. or once every day)

113. 6 mg

$$\left(9 \text{ mos} \times \frac{\overset{2}{\cancel{100}} \text{ mg}}{\underset{3}{\cancel{150} \text{ mos}}} = \frac{18 \text{ mg}}{3} = 6 \text{ mg}\right)$$

114. 23 mg

$$\left(34 \text{ lb} \times \frac{\overset{2}{\cancel{100}} \text{ mg}}{\underset{3}{\cancel{150} \text{ lb}}} = \frac{68 \text{ mg}}{3} = 22\tfrac{2}{3} \text{ mg, or about 23 mg}\right)$$

115. 80 mg

$$\left(10 \text{ yr} = 120 \text{ mos}; \ 120 \text{ mos} \times \frac{\overset{2}{\cancel{100}} \text{ mg}}{\cancel{150} \text{ mos}} = \frac{240}{3} \text{ mg} = 80 \text{ mg}\right)$$

116. 100 mg

(Anyone over 12½ years old is considered an adult.)

117. 1. 25 gtt/minute

$$\left(\frac{\overset{100}{\cancel{500} \text{ cc}}}{\underset{1}{\cancel{5} \text{ hour}}} \times \frac{\overset{1}{\cancel{15} \text{ gtt}}}{1 \text{ cc}} \times \frac{1 \text{ hour}}{\underset{4}{\cancel{60} \text{ minutes}}} = \frac{100}{4} \text{ or 25 gtt/minute}\right)$$

118. 2. 33 gtt/minute

$$\left(\frac{\overset{100}{\cancel{500} \text{ cc}}}{\underset{1}{\cancel{5} \text{ hour}}} \times \frac{\overset{1}{\cancel{20} \text{ gtt}}}{1 \text{ cc}} \times \frac{1 \text{ hour}}{\underset{3}{\cancel{60} \text{ minutes}}} = \frac{100}{3} \text{ or 3 gtt/minute}\right)$$

119. 3. 16 gtt/minute

$$\left(\frac{\overset{250}{\cancel{1500} \text{ ml}}}{\underset{4}{\cancel{24} \text{ hour}}} \times \frac{\overset{1}{\cancel{15} \text{ gtt}}}{1 \text{ cc}} \times \frac{1 \text{ hour}}{\underset{4}{\cancel{60} \text{ minutes}}} = \frac{250}{16} \text{ or 15.6} = 16 \text{ gtt/minute}\right)$$

120. 4. 25 gtt/minute

$$\left(\frac{\overset{100}{\cancel{2000} \text{ cc}}}{\underset{1}{\cancel{20} \text{ hour}}} \times \frac{\overset{1}{\cancel{15} \text{ gtt}}}{1 \text{ ml}} \times \frac{1 \text{ hour}}{\underset{4}{\cancel{60} \text{ minutes}}} = \frac{100}{4} \text{ or 25 gtt/minute}\right)$$

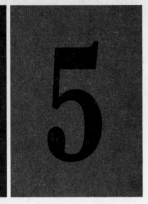

Routine Responsibilities

◆◆ In this chapter you will learn how to do the routine tasks involved in giving medications: how to order, store, and dispose of drugs; how to keep track of medication orders; how to set up medications; and how to chart medications after giving them. You will also learn how to give drugs safely by following the basic rules of medication administration.

COMPETENCIES

After studying this chapter, you should be able to

• order drugs from the pharmacy using the physician's order sheet or a pharmacy requisition.

• identify single-dose and multiple-dose packaging of drugs.

• store medicines properly as stock supplies or patient supplies in the medicine room.

• tell how a medicine cart and a medicine tray are used in giving medications.

• tell how the Kardex, medicine card, and medication record are used to communicate medication orders.

• transcribe medication orders onto the Kardex, medicine cards, and/or medication records.

• count controlled substances at the beginning of each shift and tell why this is done.

• set up medications following proper procedure.

• state the rules for giving medications and explain each one.

• fill out a proof-of-use record and tell why this is done.

• describe the patient chart and fill out related forms.

• describe the problem-oriented medical record and the subjective–objective–assessment–plan method of charting.

• follow the principles of proper charting.

• report medication errors and skipped medications on the proper forms.

VOCABULARY

ampule: a small, sealed glass container holding medication for injection; a vial

charting: keeping records of all patient care on appropriate forms

controlled substances: drugs whose use is restricted

expiration date: date after which a drug should not be used

incident report: a form used for giving information about a drug error, patient injury, or accident; also called medication error form

Kardex file: portable card file listing daily medication orders and treatments for all patients on the unit

medication error form: also called incident report

medication record: form showing routine and PRN medications ordered for a patient; each dose is checked off after it is given

medicine cards: small cards used for setting up medications when a unit-dose system is not used

medicine cart: movable unit for dispensing medications

medicine room: area where drugs are stored

nurses' notes: form for charting observations, stat and PRN medications, and special treatments given

patient chart: a permanent record of care received

patient history sheet: a form describing the development of the patient's symptoms and the course of the disease

pharmacy requisition: form on which to order supplies and medications from the pharmacy

POMR: problem-oriented medical record

proof-of-use record: form for keeping track of the administration of controlled substances; shows doses available and doses administered

routine drugs: drugs given on a regular schedule

self-terminating orders: orders for a drug to be given only until a certain date or time; also called automatic stop orders

set up: to organize the drugs for administration by arranging the proper doses on a tray or a cart

SOAP: structured plan for charting; standards for subjective–objective–assessment–plan

stock supply: a collection of drugs commonly used by patients, such as lotions, milk of magnesia, and aspirin

strip label: part of a medication label that can be torn off and placed on a reorder sheet

vial: small bottle containing one or more doses of a liquid or powdered drug for injection; an ampule

ORDERING DRUGS FROM THE PHARMACY

After a physician writes a medication order for a patient, the proper drugs must be obtained. The way this is done depends on the type of facility in which you work.

Most hospitals have a pharmacy located within the building. They may also have satellite or minipharmacies on each ward.

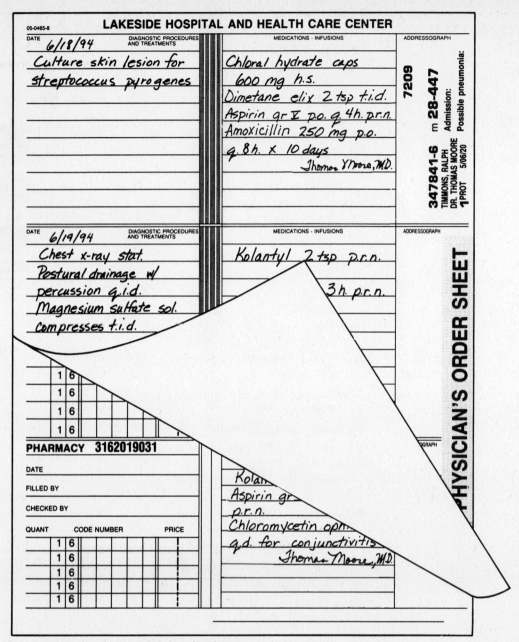

LAKESIDE HOSPITAL AND HEALTH CARE CENTER

05-0465-8

DATE 6/18/94	DIAGNOSTIC PROCEDURES AND TREATMENTS	MEDICATIONS - INFUSIONS	ADDRESSOGRAPH

Culture skin lesion for
streptococcus pyrogenes

Chloral hydrate caps
600 mg h.s.
Dimetane elix 2 tsp t.i.d.
Aspirin gr X po. q. 4h. p.r.n.
Amoxicillin 250 mg p.o.
q. 8h. x 10 days
                    Thomas Moore, M.D.

7209

347841-6   m 28-447

TIMMONS, RALPH
DR. THOMAS MOORE
1PROT   5/06/20

Admission:
Possible pneumonia:

DATE 6/19/94	DIAGNOSTIC PROCEDURES AND TREATMENTS	MEDICATIONS - INFUSIONS	ADDRESSOGRAPH

Chest x-ray stat.
Postural drainage w/
percussion q.i.d.
Magnesium sulfate sol.
compresses t.i.d.

Kolantyl 2 tsp p.r.n.

3h. p.r.n.

PHYSICIAN'S ORDER SHEET

1 6
1 6
1 6
1 6

PHARMACY   3162019031

DATE

FILLED BY

CHECKED BY

QUANT   CODE NUMBER   PRICE

1 6
1 6
1 6
1 6
1 6

Kola
Aspirin gr
p.r.n.
Chloromycetin oph
q.d. for conjunctivitis
            Thomas Moore, M.D.

Figure 5-1 Physician's order sheet and carbon for pharmacy.

Pharmacy requests can be made in several ways. The physician's order sheet usually has a second page that makes a carbon copy of the medication order (Figure 5-1). This second page can be torn out and sent to the pharmacy. It tells the pharmacist which drugs, and in which form, to send back to the ward for the patient. In some facilities, the entire patient chart is sent to the pharmacy. The chart includes the original physician's order sheet. This is the safest method of ordering drugs because the pharmacist can follow the doctor's original order in preparing the medication.

If a chart or a copy of the physician's order sheet cannot be used, the nurse must write out the drug orders on a **pharmacy requisition form** (Figure 5-2). This is sent to the pharmacist, and the orders are filled from it. There may be more than one drug order on each requisition form. When filling out a pharmacy requisition form, it is extremely important to copy all of the information correctly from the doctor's order. Be sure to fill in every item on the form. Study Figure 5-2 to see what information is included.

Using the physician's order sheet for ordering drugs is safer than using a requisition form because no copying is required. There is less chance of a medication error. When and if there is an error, it is much easier to find the source. State laws have helped to establish this single-entry ordering system because they require the order to go from the doctor directly to the pharmacy.

◆ **NOTE** ◆◆◆◆◆◆◆◆◆◆◆◆◆◆◆◆◆

State laws and agency policies regulate who may carry out the routine responsibilities in medication administration. Check the policy manual of your health facility to find out who may calculate and measure doses; set up and administer medications; transcribe medication orders; count and handle controlled substances; order, reorder, and receive drugs from the pharmacy; observe patients and chart progress; report to the physician; give patients health instruction; and so on.

In the hospital, **routine** and stat drugs are requested every day as soon as they are ordered. The pharmacy sends up medicines three times a day. Usually it sends up enough of each drug to last 8 hours. At some facilities the pharmacist checks the medicine supplies in the ward three times a day. When a patient's supply is low, the pharmacist informs the ward supervisor, and a physician can reorder the needed drugs. If the doctor's order or reorder must be taken over the phone, it is written out on a special form with two copies, one for the patient chart and one for the pharmacy. The original top sheet is mailed to the physician for signature.

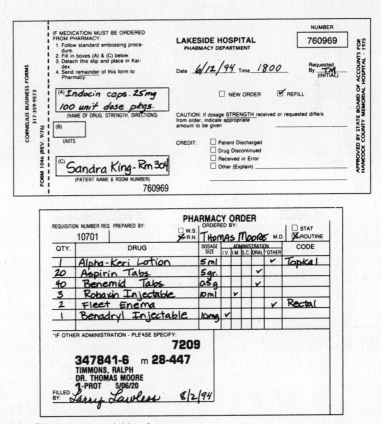

Figure 5-2 Pharmacy requisition forms.

In some hospitals, drug orders are entered into a computer, either by the doctor or by a nurse or ward clerk following the doctor's verbal or written orders.

In some facilities, drugs are reordered by sending the empty containers to the pharmacy along with appropriate requisition forms.

Some nursing homes have their own pharmacies, but most do not. They must order drugs from an outside pharmacy. The ordering system is somewhat different from the one used in hospitals. Drugs can be ordered using either a carbon copy of the physician's order sheet or a **pharmacy requisition form.** These forms are sent to the pharmacy at a certain time each day. The drugs are prepared at the pharmacy and sent back within 24 hours. When they come in, they are checked by comparing the delivery ticket with the doctor's orders.

Reorders are listed on a special reorder sheet. To make up the list, part of the original drug label called the **strip label** is pulled off of each container and pasted onto the reorder form (Figure 5-3). The form then goes to the outside pharmacy where the orders are filled.

Most drugs for nursing home patients are ordered for an indefinite period of time. In other words, they are standing orders. For that reason, drugs are ordered in large batches and are reordered only every 30–60 days.

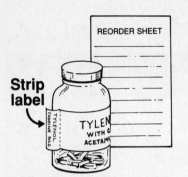

Figure 5-3 Strip label and reorder sheet.

DRUG PACKAGING

The pharmacy supplies drugs in one of two forms: single-dose packages or multiple-dose packages.

Single or Unit Dose

In single-dose or unit-dose packaging, each dose of medication is individually wrapped or bottled. Single-dose **ampules,** vials, and prefilled syringes are supplied for some parenteral medications. Each single-dose package contains the proper dose for one administration. It is labeled with the drug name, strength, expiration date, and sometimes the patient's name (Figure 5-4).

Unit-dose packaging provides the safest and most convenient means of administering medicines. The drugs require little handling and no special preparation before being taken to the patient. Unused doses can be returned to the pharmacy for credit. The individual wrappings ensure that they will not become contaminated in handling.

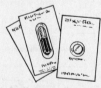 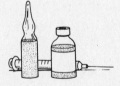

Figure 5-4 Unit-dose packages.

Multiple Dose

Many drugs are sent from the pharmacy in multiple-dose bottles or **vials** (Figure 5-5). The person who is to administer the drug must measure and pour out single doses of liquid medications or count out tablets or capsules from a bottle. Because these drugs require more handling, there is more chance for error than with unit-dose packages. Unused drugs from multiple-dose containers cannot be credited to the patient's account. They are destroyed in the pharmacy because they may have been contaminated.

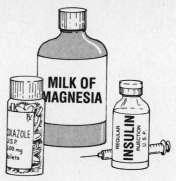

Figure 5-5 Multiple-dose packages.

STORAGE AND DISPOSAL OF DRUGS

Medicine Room

All medications are stored in a special area, usually located behind the nurses' station of each unit. This is known as the **medicine room** (Figure 5-6). It is open only to authorized personnel.

The medicine room contains a sink, a refrigerator, and a number of cabinets. The refrigerator is needed because some drugs must be stored in a cool place; otherwise, they lose their effectiveness. Drugs that need refrigeration are so labeled. Among them are insulin, antibiotics, suppositories, eyedrops, and tetanus vaccine.

There is a special cabinet in the medicine room for controlled substances. It is kept locked so that the use of these restricted drugs can be monitored.

Another cabinet may hold **stock supply** drugs, or drugs commonly used by many patients. Some stock supply drugs are also kept in the refrigerator. Drugs like aspirin, milk of magnesia, penicillin, lotions, and emergency medications are often part of the stock supply. Because of the new unit-dose system, stock supplies are not as common as they used to be.

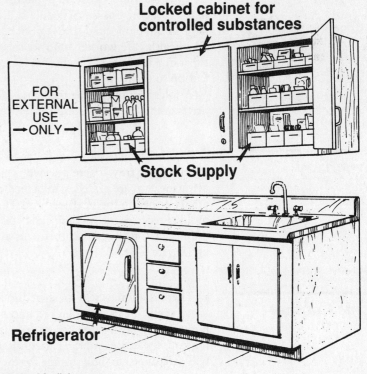

Figure 5-6 Medicine room.

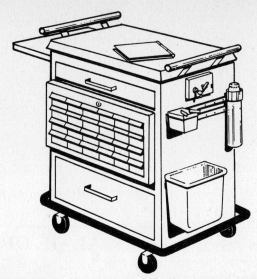

Figure 5-7   Medicine cart.

Cabinets in the medicine room should be kept closed at all times. Many drugs break down if they are exposed to light. Drugs that are for external use only are always kept in separate cabinets or compartments.

Keep the medicine room and refrigerator clean and tidy at all times. This is vital in helping to prevent medication errors.

Medicine Cart

For convenience, doses of routine drugs are often stored in a **medicine cart**. It is kept locked when not in use. This cart has drawers marked off for different patients. A supply of unit-dose packages is kept in each patient's drawer. When it is time for a dose to be given, the cart can be wheeled from room to room. The medications are then dispensed right out of the drawers (Figure 5-7).

Within the drawers, sections may be divided and labeled to hold routine medications, bedtime medications, and PRN medications. A special locked drawer in the cart contains the Schedule II, III, and IV drugs. (Schedule II drugs must be kept in double-locked drawers. Schedule III and IV drugs may be kept there.) The health care worker unlocks this drawer only when a dose of a controlled substance is needed. The drawer is relocked immediately, before giving the medication to the patient.

A folder on top of the medicine cart contains the paperwork that tells which drugs are to be administered at which times.

Medicine Tray

Another way of carrying drugs from room to room at administration time is the medicine tray. There are two types of trays. One is a flat tray on which the medicine cups are placed, with a medicine card next to each of them. (These cards are described in the next section.) The other is a Styrofoam or plastic tray with molded recesses for holding cups and medicine cards. The molded tray is better than the flat tray because the cards and cups cannot move about and get mixed up (Figure 5-8).

Medicine Cabinet

There is another way to store medications in addition to the medicine room. It is a medicine cabinet, locked and hung on the wall. The nurse caring for the patient each day has the key to open it. This storage system saves time and effort for both the nurse and the patient. Regarding narcotics, most likely your agency will determine narcotic storage for the patients. These would be narcotics that do not have to be accounted for, as in the stock supply.

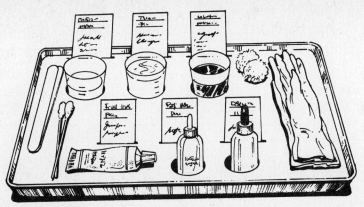

Figure 5-8 Medicine tray.

Disposing of Unused Drugs

Unused doses of medications should never be returned to stock supply bottles. Discard the unused doses in the proper manner. Each health facility has its own policy regarding drug disposal. Usually the drugs must be returned to the pharmacy. In some cases, they must go to a certain person or storage area. They are then held until there is a batch of drugs to return to the pharmacy. The disposal of controlled substances must be witnessed by another staff member. It must then be noted on the proper form.

KEEPING TRACK OF MEDICATION ORDERS

Whenever more than one patient is being cared for, it is necessary to keep track of which patient is supposed to get which medicine at what time. In a ward of 20 patients, some of whom are to receive several drugs, careful preparation is needed to keep their medications straight. Medical facilities and nursing homes have various ways of handling this problem. Three common aids—the Kardex file, medicine cards, and the medication record—are helpful.

Kardex

The **Kardex file** is a handy means of communication among doctors and the nursing staff (Figure 5-9). It consists of a set of index cards in a portable file. A card for each patient gives up-to-date information about medications and treatments ordered. Each time new orders are given, the old ones are erased and the new ones penciled in. The Kardex is a quick reference when any member of the health team needs to know about a patient's daily course of treatment. Health workers can use the Kardex to help organize their own work day. They can also use it to **set up** medications. This involves organizing the drugs for administration by arranging the proper doses on a tray or a cart.

Medicine Cards

Medicine cards are another aid in keeping track of medications (Figure 5-10, pg. 99). They are not used as often today as in the past because the unit-dose system has cut down on the need for them. Where they are still used, information is transcribed or copied onto a set of medicine cards from the Kardex. One medicine card is written out for each type of drug that a patient is to receive. Each card states the patient's name; room and bed number; name of the drug, dose, route, and time at which the drug is to be given; and other notes in regard to specific medications. Sometimes the card also includes the signature of the nurse or clerk who copied the information from the Kardex.

Medicine cards are kept in the medicine room and picked up each hour just before setting up the drug tray.

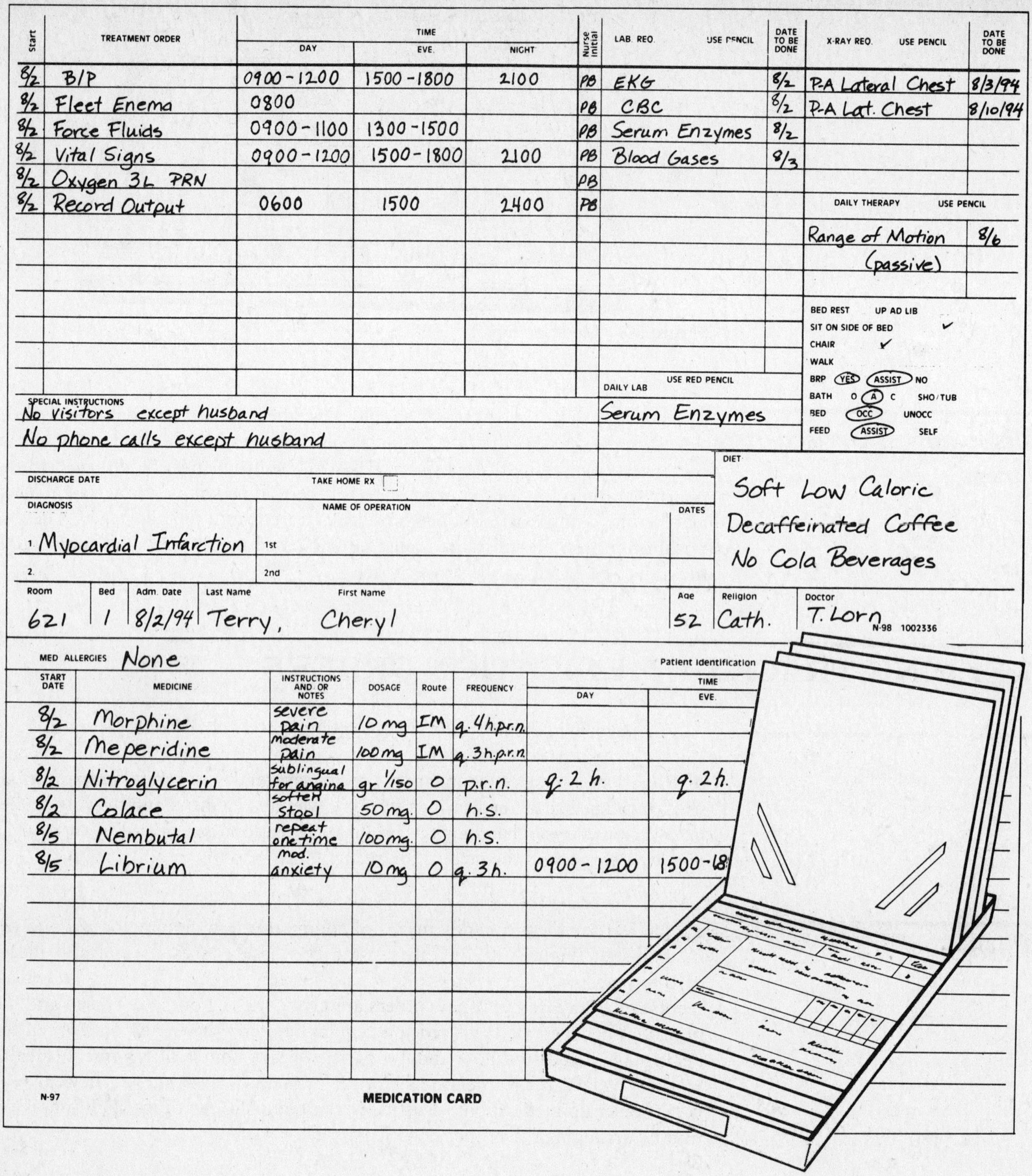

Start	TREATMENT ORDER	TIME DAY	EVE.	NIGHT	Nurse initial	LAB. REQ. USE PENCIL	DATE TO BE DONE	X-RAY REQ. USE PENCIL	DATE TO BE DONE
8/2	B/P	0900-1200	1500-1800	2100	PB	EKG	8/2	P-A Lateral Chest	8/3/94
8/2	Fleet Enema	0800			PB	CBC	8/2	P-A Lat. Chest	8/10/94
8/2	Force Fluids	0900-1100	1300-1500		PB	Serum Enzymes	8/2		
8/2	Vital Signs	0900-1200	1500-1800	2100	PB	Blood Gases	8/3		
8/2	Oxygen 3L PRN				PB				
8/2	Record Output	0600	1500	2400	PB			DAILY THERAPY USE PENCIL	
								Range of Motion	8/6
								(passive)	

BED REST   UP AD LIB
SIT ON SIDE OF BED   ✓
CHAIR   ✓
WALK
BRP (YES) (ASSIST) NO
BATH O (A) C   SHO/TUB
BED (OCC) UNOCC
FEED (ASSIST) SELF

SPECIAL INSTRUCTIONS
No visitors except husband
No phone calls except husband

DAILY LAB   USE RED PENCIL
Serum Enzymes

DISCHARGE DATE   TAKE HOME RX ☐

DIET
Soft Low Caloric
Decaffeinated Coffee
No Cola Beverages

DIAGNOSIS   NAME OF OPERATION   DATES
1. Myocardial Infarction   1st
2.   2nd

Room	Bed	Adm. Date	Last Name	First Name	Age	Religion	Doctor
621	1	8/2/94	Terry,	Cheryl	52	Cath.	T. Lorn N-98 1002336

MED ALLERGIES None   Patient Identification

START DATE	MEDICINE	INSTRUCTIONS AND OR NOTES	DOSAGE	Route	FREQUENCY	TIME DAY	EVE.
8/2	Morphine	severe pain	10 mg	IM	q. 4h. p.r.n.		
8/2	Meperidine	moderate pain	100 mg	IM	q. 3h. p.r.n.		
8/2	Nitroglycerin	sublingual for angina	gr 1/150	O	p.r.n.	q. 2 h.	q. 2 h.
8/2	Colace	soften stool	50 mg.	O	h.s.		
8/5	Nembutal	repeat one time	100 mg.	O	h.s.		
8/5	Librium	mod. anxiety	10 mg	O	q. 3h.	0900-1200	1500-18

N-97   **MEDICATION CARD**

Figure 5-9 Kardex.

If the information on a medicine card seems unclear to you, be sure to recheck the Kardex and the physician's order sheet. A mistake may have been made in copying this information. Never try to read through a card that has medicine spilled on it. You may make a medication error. Go back to the patient's chart and the Kardex and make a new medicine card. However, be sure that you copy the information correctly onto the new card. If you need more help, consult the nurse in charge or the drug references on your unit.

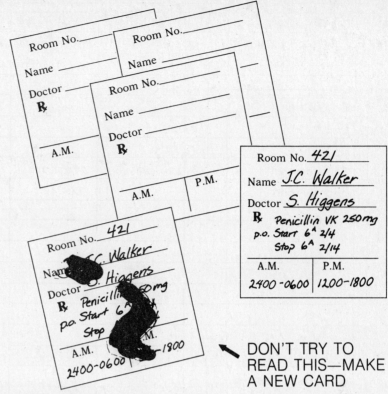

Figure 5-10 Medicine cards.

DON'T TRY TO READ THIS—MAKE A NEW CARD

Medication Record ◆◆

The **medication record** is a convenient way of keeping track when more than one drug is being administered to a particular patient every day. It is especially helpful when several drugs are to be given at different times. The name of each drug is written down once on a patient's medication record (Figures 5-11 and 5-12, pp. 100–101). There are separate sections for routine and PRN medications. The amount, strength, and route are also noted.

If a drug is to be given regularly, a complete schedule is written out of all the administration times for that drug. Then, each time a dose is administered, the health care worker checks off the time it was given and initials it. The full name of each person dispensing medications is listed somewhere on the sheet. This is done so that the initials can be identified, if needed.

The medication record is prepared by the clerk, pharmacist, or other health care worker as drugs are ordered. The nurse then checks the form against the doctor's order and signs it. Medication records for all patients may be kept in a special folder on the medicine cart. Or they may be kept in individual patient charts.

Self-Terminating Orders ◆◆

Self-terminating or automatic stop orders mean that the drug is to be given only until a certain date or time. When this type of order is copied from the physician's order sheet, the nurse or clerk makes a special note or mark on the Kardex, medicine cards, or medication record. This shows the date and time when the drug should stop being given. In Figures 5-11 and 5-12, the orders for chloromycetin show examples of such notes. When that time comes, the nurse or clerk will notify the patient's doctor that the order has terminated. If the doctor decides that the patient needs to continue receiving the drug, a new order will be written. Remember that automatic stop orders usually cover antibiotics, narcotics, corticosteroids, anticoagulants, and barbiturates.

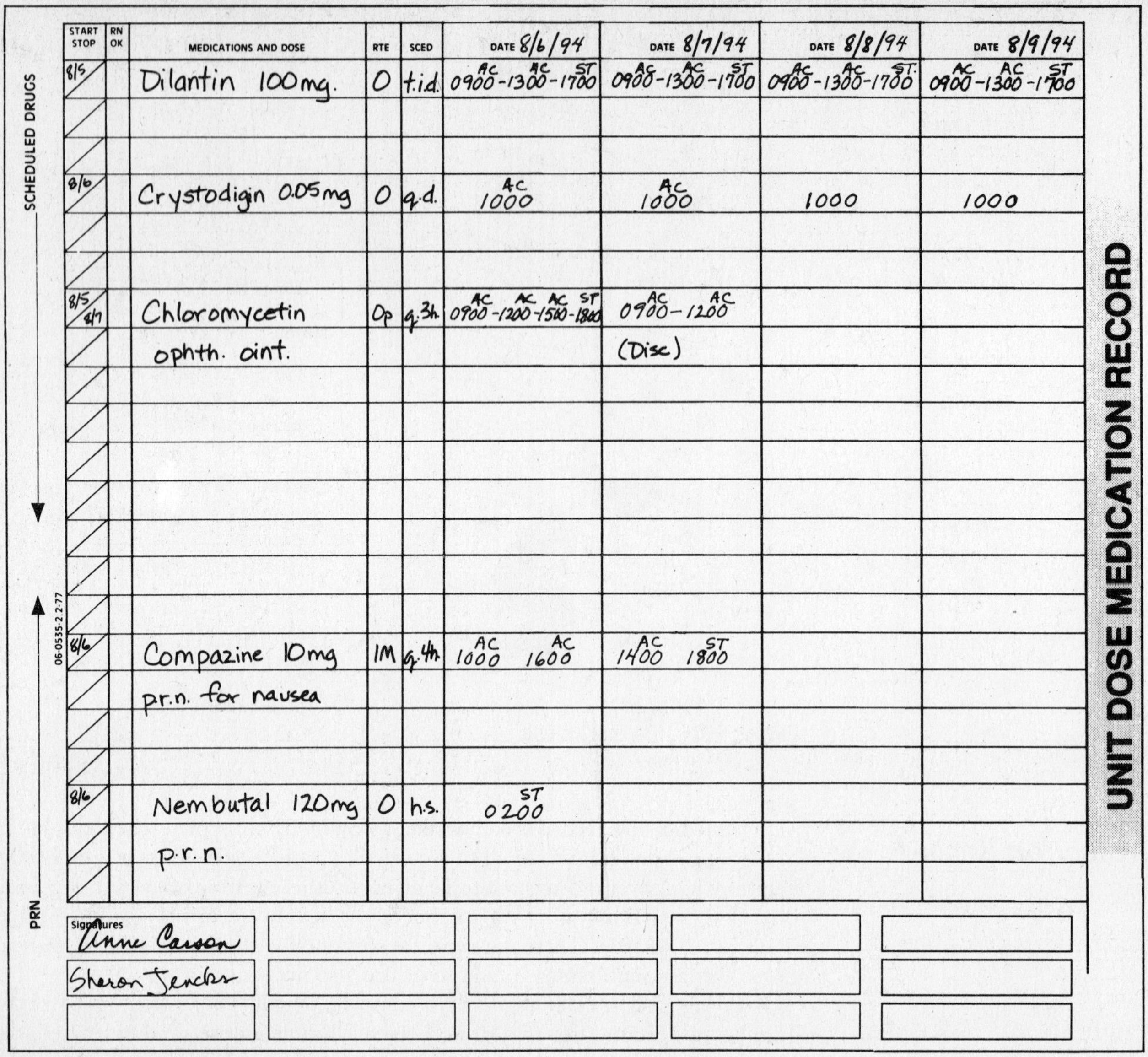

START STOP	RN OK	MEDICATIONS AND DOSE	RTE	SCED	DATE 8/6/94	DATE 8/7/94	DATE 8/8/94	DATE 8/9/94
8/5		Dilantin 100 mg.	O	t.i.d.	AC AC ST 0900-1300-1700	AC AC ST 0900-1300-1700	AC AC ST 0900-1300-1700	AC AC ST 0900-1300-1700
8/6		Crystodigin 0.05 mg	O	q.d.	AC 1000	AC 1000	1000	1000
8/5 4/7		Chloromycetin ophth. oint.	Op	q.3h.	AC AC AC ST 0900-1200-1500-1800	AC AC 0900-1200 (Disc)		
8/6		Compazine 10 mg pr.n. for nausea	IM	q.4h.	AC 1000 AC 1600	AC 1400 ST 1800		
8/6		Nembutal 120 mg p.r.n.	O	h.s.	ST 0200			
Signatures		Anne Carson						
		Sharon Jencks						

Margin labels: SCHEDULED DRUGS / PRN / 06-0535-2 2-77 / UNIT DOSE MEDICATION RECORD

Figure 5-11 Medication record form.

Controlled Substances

Controlled substances are drugs whose use is restricted. This group of drugs includes narcotics, stimulants, and depressants (see Chapter 1).

Because of legal restrictions, these medications must be counted or measured at the beginning of each shift. As the shift changes, the person coming off duty and the person coming on duty do the counting and measuring together. They record the quantity of each controlled substance on forms for that purpose. They then sign a special form so that there is a record of who counted the drugs on each shift (Figure 5-13). If the count is found to be incorrect at a later shift, the error can be traced to the proper persons.

Controlled substances are sometimes sent to the ward in special containers that allow easy counting. They are packaged in either single doses or multiple doses. The packages are given a special seal at the pharmacy. Only medications in packages on which the seal is broken (showing that they have been used) need to be measured and counted.

Each time a controlled substance is administered to a patient from the stock supply, the health worker must sign a **proof-of-use record,** such as the one shown in Figure 5-14 on page 102. Each health facility has its own form for this pur-

MEDICATION RECORD																																

Family Name: Shrock   **First Name:** Tammy   **Middle Name:** Anne   **Month:** Sept   **Year:** 1994   **Room No.** 517   **Bed No.** 1   **Admission No.** 874321

Attending Physician: N. Morris   **Supervising Nurse:** P. T. Brown

MEDICATIONS	Hour	1	2	3	4	5	6	7	8	9	10	11	12	13	14	15	16	17	18	19	20	21	22	23	24	25	26	27	28	29	30	31
Dilantin 100 mg p.o.	0900	LE	LE	LE	AW	AW	LE																										
t.i.d.	1300	LE	LE	LE	AW	AW	(LE)																										
	1700	CS	CS	CS	NF	NF																											
Chloromycetin ophth.	0900	LE	LE	LE	AW	AW	LE				X																						
oint. q.i.d.	1200	LE	LE	LE	AW	AW	LE				X																						
	1500	CS	CS	(CS)	CS	NF	NF				X																						
	1800	CS	CS	CS	CS	NF	NF				X																						
							last dose 1200 (D)																										

INSULIN TYPE	Hour Given	Amount Given	U 16	U 16	U 16	U 16	U 17	U 17																									
NPH	0600																																	
CODE	R-Refused D-Discontinued O-Ordered	Sugar	N	N	N	+	+	N																									
		Acetone	N	N	N	+	+	+																									

Initial medications and identify initials below with signature

NURSES	INITIALS	SIGNATURES	NURSES	INITIALS	SIGNATURES	NURSES	INITIALS	SIGNATURES
A.M. Nurse	LE	Lorna Emmett	P.M. Nurse	CS	Carl Simmer	Night Nurse	KB	Karen Black
A.M. Relief	AW	Alice Wright	P.M. Relief	NF	Halma Francis	Night Relief	TT	Tillie Tate

FORM NH-302   PHYSICIANS RECORD CO., BERWYN, ILLINOIS · PRINTED IN U.S.A.

Figure 5-12 Medication record form.

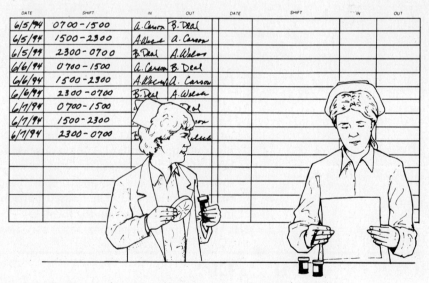

DATE	SHIFT	IN	OUT	DATE	SHIFT	IN	OUT
6/5/94	0700–1500	A. Carson	B. Deal				
6/5/94	1500–2300	A. West	A. Carson				
6/5/94	2300–0700	B. Deal	A. West				
6/6/94	0700–1500	A. Carson	B. Deal				
6/6/94	1500–2300	A. West	A. Carson				
6/6/94	2300–0700	B. Deal	A. West				
6/7/94	0700–1500						
6/7/94	1500–2300						
6/7/94	2300–0700						

Figure 5-13 Count controlled substances at beginning of each shift.

CHECK ONE	NARCOTIC/BARBITURATE PROOF OF USE RECORD

CHECK ONE
- ☐ DO NOT REISSUE
- ☑ REISSUE
- ☐ MED DISCONTINUED
- ☐ PAT. DISCHARGED
- ☐ OTHER

NARCOTIC/BARBITURATE PROOF OF USE RECORD

LAKESIDE HOSPITAL

RETURNED BY: *Greg Storms, Pharm. Aide* DATE: 8/11/94

RECEIVED BY: *P. Long, R.N.* DATE: 8/11/94

ALL PREPS LOST, DESTROYED OR UNACCOUNTED FOR MUST BE EXPLAINED.

NO	DATE	TIME	PATIENT	BED	AM'T mgs	PHYSICIAN	ADMIN. BY	AMOUNT & WITNESS
25	8/11/94	1600	Carol McCullum	921	100 mg	T. Mann	P. Long	
24	8/12/94	0800	Shirley Dugan	912	75 mg	P. Zipp	g. Caf	25mg/g. Jones
23	8/14/94	1400	Ricky Hornett	924	100 mg	D. Perkins	C. Kelly	
22	8/19/94	1300	Robert Lane	916	100 mg	P. Zipp	C. Kelly	
21	8/21/94	0630	Kelly Radner	910	50 mg	C. Ruff	P. Long	50mg/H. Holly
20								
19								
18								
17								
16								
15								
14								
13								
12								
11								
10								
9								
8								
7								
6								
5								
4								
3								
2								
1								

USE LINES BELOW FOR CORRECTION OF ERRORS WHEN APPLICABLE

ISSUED TO:

Unit C

UNIT OR PATIENT NAME & BED NO.

ISSUED BY: *M. Cheung, R.PH*

RECEIVED BY: *Greg Storms, Pharm aide*

SERIAL NO. 461 NO. ISSUED 25 DATE 8/11/94

DRUG NAME	STRENGTH	FORM	SIZE
Demerol	100mg	ampuls	2 ml

Figure 5-14 Proof-of-use record for controlled substances.

pose. The form usually shows the number of doses sent to the ward stock supply from the pharmacy. As each dose is used, the date, time, patient, room number, amount given, physician, and person administering the dose must be written down. If a dose less than the prepared individual dose is given, the amount actually given is noted. The unused portion must be destroyed in front of a witness, who must also sign the form.

ROLE OF COMPUTERS

Computers play a large role in our society. When you begin working in a hospital, you may find computers at the nurses' station (Figure 5-15). In some

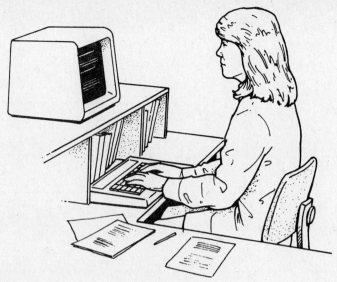

Figure 5-15 Inputting drug administration data.

hospitals, much of the drug ordering and record keeping are done by computer. (You will be trained on the job for those computer-related activities, but a computer course will greatly increase your understanding of the system and how it operates.)

Computer systems used in different hospitals vary, and improvements are being made all the time. But let's look at some kinds of information that can be processed by computer.

Let us take the example of John Smith, who has already been hospitalized for a while. His current medications of insulin and *Lanoxin* have already been entered into the system. Now his doctor wishes to add a PRN order for codeine. The physician can do this in the usual way by writing a medication order. The nurse or unit clerk then enters it into the computer system as a new medical order (Figure 5-16a). A label for this prescription is then printed out in the pharmacy (Figure 5-16b). The prescription is filled and brought to the floor.

Based on the information entered, the computer will print out at regular intervals, usually hourly, the medications scheduled for a particular floor (Figure 5-16c). Also at regular intervals, the computer will print a listing of unscheduled or miscellaneous drugs (Figure 5-16d). When the drugs on either of these printouts are given, that information is entered. Figure 5-16e shows all the charting done for a specific patient, John Smith, over the past 24 hours.

Whether you chart information in writing in the patient's record or enter it into the computer, you must be very careful and accurate. And be sure to do your recording when this is supposed to be done.

SETTING UP MEDICATIONS

The medications are ordered by the physician, requested from the pharmacy, and stored in the proper area. Now comes the time when you, the giver of medications, must be most alert—setting up medications. Setting up medications means taking information given on the Kardex, medication record, or medicine card and preparing an actual dose of medication for a patient. You will be setting up several drugs at a time, and you must be aware of all of the possibilities

a
```
50   -0003-01      UNITED HOSPITAL
07/28/94  2:13 P.M.                                    PAGE 001
                        NEW MEDICAL ORDERS
SMITH J.          M  40   123456789012              ADM:07/11/94
  BED:C501-D  N/S: 5C        SERV: INT   -JONES T. MD
  PRIMARY DIAGNOSIS: ILL
  ENTERED BY: BROWN KATHY E      H  ENTERED FOR: NURSE
  TIME ENTERED: 07/28/94   2:13 PM
  ORDER TYPE: WRITTEN ORDER


     CODEINE TAB 15MG, 1,PO, Q4H, PRN PAIN, (KLD).

            NOTED BY NURSE: _____

                  LAST PAGE
```

b
```
                              PHRMI-0004
   123456-7-89012  07/28/94     123456-7-89012  07/28/94  2:13 PM
   SMITH J.        C501-D        SMITH J.   40 M   C501-D
   CODEINE TAB 15MG 1,PO         CODEINE TAB 15MG 1,PO Q4H PRN PAIN
                                 . (# 28) .

        BROWN KATHY E   H=4 KL         BROWN KATHY E    H=4 KL
        ENTERED FOR: NURSE             ENTERED FOR NURSE

   FILLED BY:_____     ALLERGIES: NONE REPORTED


   NAME: SMITH J.
   ROOM #: C501-D
   PATIENT#: 123456-7-89012
   DATE: 07/28/94
   ITEM# 43011002
   DESC. CODEINE TAB 15MG


   AMOUNT_____._____      FILLED BY_____
   _*_
```

c
```
50    -0004          UNITED HOSPITAL
     09:00 AM SCHEDULED MEDICATIONS DUE 5C    07-29-94
                                   ISSUED 02:01 PM 07/28/94


C517-W  BB BBBBBB PREADMIT                     GIV NGIV

ALDACTONE TAB 25MG, 1,PO, Q1H, (06/10/94) 07 AM-..), (KG).   --- ---

C501-D SMITH J.                                GIV NGIV

INSULIN REGULAR U-100 15 UNITS, INSULIN LENTE U-100 36
UNITS, SC, DAILY, (07/18/94 09AM-..), (KLD).                 --- ---

LANOXIN LANOXIN TAB 0.25 MG, 1,PO, DAILY, (07/18/94 09AM-..)
, (KLD).                                                     --- ---
_*_
```

d
```
50    -0004          UNITED HOSPITAL
           UNSCHED&MISC MEDS   5C    07/28/94
                              ISSUED 02:14 PM 07/28/94


C501-D SMITH J.
                                               GIV NGIV

LIDOCAINE INJ XYLOCAINE IV INJ 75 MG,BOLUS IV PUSH , NOW--
ALREADY GIVEN FOLLOWED WITH LIDOCAINE DRIP, (KLD).           --- ---

CODEINE TAB 15MG, 1,PO, Q4H, PRN PAIN, (KLD).                --- ---
_*_
```

e
```
                         UNITED HOSPITAL
07/28/94  2:17 PM                 PAGE 001
QAT$$P


= = = = = = = = = = = = = = = =
SMITH J.              M 40 C501-D          = = = = = = = =
123456-7-89012 ADM: 07/11/94               PATIENT RECORD
DX: ILL                                    = = = = = = = =
= = = = = = = = = = = = = = = =

     DATE ENTERED DURING:   07/28/ 12:00 MN TO 2:17 PM
= = = = = = = = = = = = = = = = = = = = = = = = = = = = =

MEDICATIONS:
INSULIN REGULAR U-100 15 UNITS, INSULIN LENTE U- 100 36 UNITS,
   07/28  9:00 AM SC,GIV,INJ SITE:, RM ARM          BROWN KATHY E    H
CODEINE TAB 15MG
   07/28  2:00 PM 2, PO, GIV,FOR,PAIN,LT,UPPER,BACK   BROWN KATHY E    H
LANOXIN TAB 0.25 MG
   07/28  9:00 AM 2,PO,NOT GIV,LANOXIN,BECAUSE:,
            LETHARGIC                               BROWN KATHY E    H
                  ** END OF REPORT **

                  LAST PAGE
```

Figure 5-16 Examples of computer-generated forms and information.

for error. Here are some guidelines to help you prepare a medicine tray or drug cart for your rounds.

1. *Clear your mind of all thoughts except getting your medications set up properly.* Do not try to carry on a conversation with someone while you work; the task at hand needs your full attention.

2. *Before handling any medications, think about cleanliness and the possibility of spreading germs.* Germs can be transmitted to patients on tablets and other medications, so follow aseptic procedure (see a fuller discussion in Chapter 6). Wash your hands before touching any drug product. Try not to touch them at all, but pour them directly into paper or plastic medicine cups. Never give a pill that has fallen on the floor; throw it out. Do not cough or sneeze on the medications. Keep unit doses sealed until you are ready to give them.

3. *When you take the medication from the storage area, check the expiration date and notice if there is any change in color, smell, or texture.* Any physical change may mean that the drug has lost its effectiveness, perhaps because of improper storage or extremes of temperature. If you note anything unusual about the appearance of a drug, do not give it to the patient. Send it back to the pharmacy for replacement.

4. *Setting up is the time when you need to decide whether you must calculate a dose.* You will notice whether the pharmacist's order is in a unit of measurement different from that of the physician's order. At this point the skills you learned in Chapter 4 will come in handy. Remember to use conversion tables and have your work checked if you have any doubts at all. If you need to divide a tablet, place it on a clean paper towel or tissue. Use a knife edge to press down hard on the scored part to make a quick, clean break.

5. *When you pour liquid medication from a bottle, pour it on the side away from the label.* Then if there is a drip from the mouth of the bottle, it will not smudge the label. The label is very important in helping you choose the right drug next time your patient needs it. Hold the measuring container at eye level so that you can see that you are getting the exact amount. The liquid will tend to curve up along the sides of the container; the lowest part of the curve should be even with the marked measure you want (Figure 5-17).

6. *After removing the desired dose from a bottle, recap the bottle tightly.* Then replace the bottle in the cabinet, refrigerator, or cart, taking care to keep the medication area neatly arranged.

7. *Decide whether the medication is to be mixed with a liquid or food.* Drugs are sometimes mixed with food or drink to hide their taste. Tablets may be crushed and capsules opened and mixed to make them easier for a patient to swallow. If the doctor's order does not give special instructions, check the package insert.

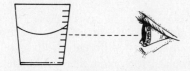

Figure 5-17 Measure liquid at eye level.

Drugs cannot be mixed with just any liquid. Some drugs are broken down by acids and others by alkalis, so the correct juice or other liquid must be selected. For example, fruit juices are acid, whereas milk is alkali. Some possible liquids with which medications may be taken are orange juice, apple juice, lemonade, cranberry juice, grape juice, milk, soup, cocoa, and coffee. Applesauce is a common choice when drugs must be mixed with food. If you do mix a medication with liquid or food, do not let the mixture stand for a long time. Give it to the patient immediately.

Further guidelines for setting up are included in the "five rights" of medication administration discussed in the next section.

RULES FOR GIVING MEDICATIONS: THE FIVE RIGHTS

The rules for giving medications are the same no matter who is giving them. Special problems and situations may exist, and individual answers are needed for them. But the basic rules and regulations never change. They are:

- Give the medicine to the **right patient**
- Give the **right drug**
- Give the **right dose**
- Give the medicine by the **right route**
- Give the medicine at the **right time**

Right Patient

Always identify the patient in some way. Make absolutely certain that you know who the patient is. Read the identification wristband that all hospital patients wear. Ask patients their names or greet a patient by name and observe the response. (This is not foolproof, however.) Get the nurse in charge to help you identify a patient, if necessary.

Check the patient's name against the name on the medicine card or medication record each time you administer medication.

Right Drug

Give only medicine that you have prepared. Give drugs only from labeled containers. Keep unit-dose packages wrapped until ready to use so the label stays with the medication. Read the label three times as you prepare the medicine (Figure 5-18):

1. As you take it from the shelf or drawer where it is stored.

2. As you pour or measure the drug.

3. As you replace the bottle or package from which you measured or poured the drug.

Be aware of the different names for the same drug—the generic name and various product names. Also be aware that very different drugs can have very similar names. *Orinase* and *Ornade,* for example, might be mistaken for each other, but one is for diabetes and the other is for a stuffy nose. This means that you should notice very carefully the spelling of the drug's name and be sure to verify an order if the handwriting is unclear.

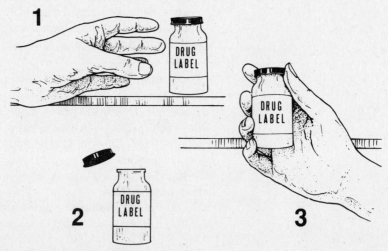

Figure 5-18 Read the label three times.

Know the abbreviation for the different dosage forms.

Recheck any medicine that the patient feels is wrong. Be sure that the label corresponds to the name of the drug written on the medicine card or medication record. And recheck to see that you have the right patient!

Right Dose

Read the package insert. It tells how to dilute or mix medications, if necessary. Also, read the package label carefully to make sure that the drug is of proper strength.

Know the correct dosage symbols and abbreviations. Use properly marked measuring containers: a minim glass for minims, medicine glasses marked with metric or apothecaries' units, and a medicine dropper if drops are ordered. If you must calculate a medicine dose, double-check your work. Recheck any drug dose that the patient feels is wrong.

Be sure that the amount the patient receives matches the amount stated on the medicine card or chart. Stay with each patient until he or she takes the medicine.

Help weak patients take medication to be sure they get the full amount.

Open capsules (except delayed-release capsules) or crush large tablets for those who have difficulty swallowing.

Right Route

Always write the route on the medicine card or medication record. Package inserts, drug references, and the patient chart can give you information about the right route. Call the nurse in charge if you still have questions after checking these references.

Know the correct abbreviations for the routes.

Be aware of factors or changes in the patient's condition that would affect the route of administration. For example, the rectal or parenteral route probably makes more sense for a patient who is vomiting than the oral route. Have the doctor write a different order when these changes arise.

Right Time

Know the correct abbreviations for times of administration.

Check the medication record or medicine card for the correct time to give a medication.

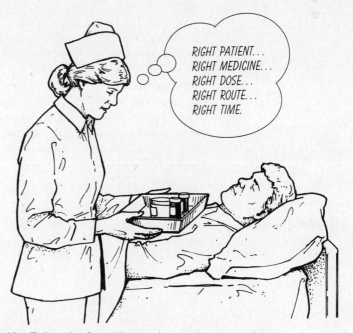

Figure 5-19   Follow the five rights to give medications safely.

Give the drug as close as possible to the stated time.

Never leave a drug at the patient's bedside unless ordered by the doctor.

Organize your work time at the beginning of each shift so that you can get medications to each patient on schedule. Review all of the day's nursing activities and your own duties. Plan accordingly, taking into account the times when patients are to receive medications (Figure 5-19).

Check whether an oral drug should be taken on an empty stomach or with food. Drugs to be taken on an empty stomach should be given 1 hour before meals or 2 hours afterward. Drugs to be taken on a full stomach should be given immediately before, with, or after a meal.

CHARTING MEDICATIONS

Any time a patient is given some form of treatment, such as medication, a record is kept of that treatment. Special problems or circumstances are also written down, such as new symptoms, the patient's own statements, laboratory tests performed, and so on. All of the events in the course of a patient's treatment are written down in the **patient chart**, which is a permanent record of care received.

The chart is an important document. First, it is a form of communication among the patient, doctor, and other members of the health care team. The patient chart is also a legal document. It is the official record of the care given to a patient. The patient or the patient's family may question the quality of treatment. The health facility can evaluate the situation by referring to the chart. If there is a lawsuit, the chart can be used in court to decide whether the patient received good or bad care. The chart is taken as proof of the care the patient received.

The chart may also be used by researchers to study certain diseases or drugs. It may serve as a teaching aid for medical students. Or it may be used to gather facts and figures about the overall performance of a certain health facility.

For all of these reasons, it is important for you to learn how to write down the necessary information on a patient chart. This is called charting.

First, you should know that not all charts look alike. Different health facilities have their own forms for keeping records. The traditional patient chart consists of a collection of different forms (Figure 5-20). Each form is filled out separately by a different member of the health care team. Individual staff members chart the problems for which they are responsible and the treatment or care that they give. Other team members refer to these specific reports as needed.

The traditional patient chart contains a form you have already seen: the physician's order sheet. This is filled out by the patient's doctor. It contains orders for tests, procedures, and drugs to treat the patient's condition. The doctor also fills out a **patient history sheet**, describing the patient's medical problems in more detail. Various other forms are used to record such things as laboratory tests, x-rays, reports of specialists, and the patient's progress. Two forms that you will deal with in administering medications are the medication record and the nurses' notes.

Medication Record

You learned what the medication record is in an earlier section. Here you will learn how to chart after the medication has been given. The following facts must be included on the medication record:

- Name of the drug
- Strength and/or amount of the drug
- Times at which the drug is to be given
- Route by which the drug is given
- Initials of the health worker who administered the drug

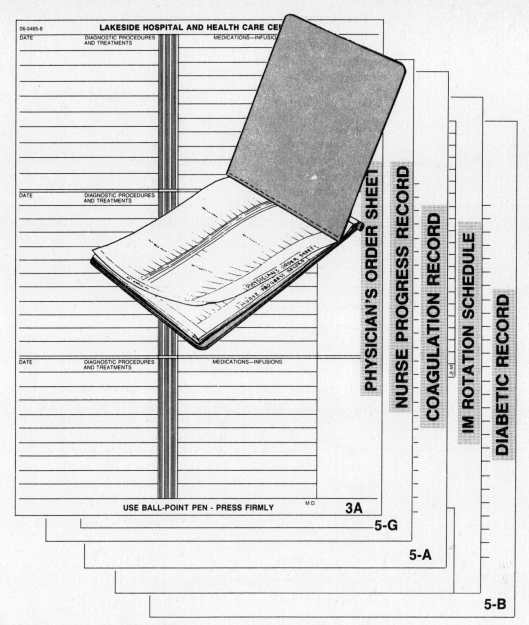

Figure 5-20 Patient chart and traditional forms.

For routine medications, most of this information has been written out ahead of time. Only your initials need to be charted each time a drug is administered. Look back at Figures 5-11 and 5-12 to see two different ways of charting on medication records.

In case a dose of medicine is not given at a scheduled time, you should indicate that fact on the chart. Usually this is done by circling the skipped time on the medication record and initialing it. You should also explain why the drug was not given on the nurses' notes.

If the medication record has a section for PRN medications, you will need to chart both the time of administration and your initials. If there is no place to chart PRN medications, you should chart them on the nurses' notes.

Nurses' Notes

The form known as **nurses' notes** is called by several names, including progress notes and nurses' progress notes. It is used by the nurse to chart observations of the patient and nursing care provided (Figure 5-21). Stat medications and sometimes PRN medications are also charted on the nurses' notes.

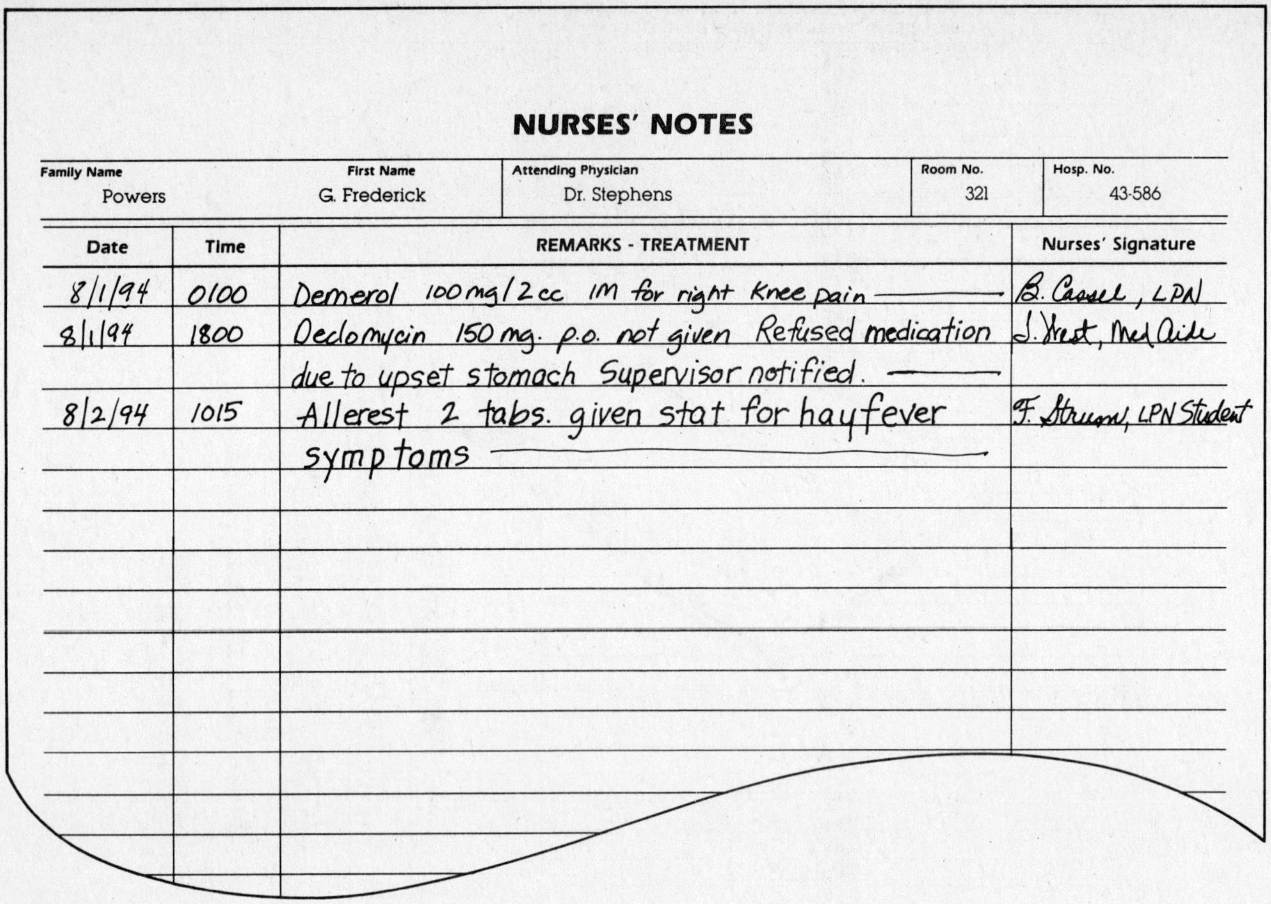

NURSES' NOTES

Family Name	First Name	Attending Physician		Room No.	Hosp. No.
Powers	G. Frederick	Dr. Stephens		321	43-586

Date	Time	REMARKS - TREATMENT	Nurses' Signature
8/1/94	0100	Demerol 100 mg/2 cc IM for right knee pain ————	B. Cassel, LPN
8/1/94	1800	Declomycin 150 mg. p.o. not given Refused medication due to upset stomach Supervisor notified. ———	J. Hest, Med Aide
8/2/94	1015	Allerest 2 tabs. given stat for hayfever symptoms ———————	F. Strum, LPN Student

Figure 5-21   Nurses' notes.

The following information must be charted in the nurses' notes each time a stat medication is given:

- Name of the drug
- Strength and/or amount of the drug administered
- Route
- Time of administration
- Results of checking vital signs (blood pressure, temperature, respiration, pulse) if required for specific drugs
- Any other special information regarding the drug or the patient (e.g., problems in getting the patient to take the drug, unusual reactions)
- Signature (first initial and last name) and title of the person who administered the drug

In addition to recording stat medications, the form includes other information. Any time you notice something unusual with any medication, you should chart it on the nurses' notes. You should also make a note on the nurses' notes any time a scheduled medication is not given. The second entry in Figure 5-21 shows a case like this.

The *POMR*

Many hospitals and other health facilities use a chart called the **POMR** (problem-oriented medical record). In this system the chart is organized according to a numbered list of problems (Figure 5-22). All health team members chart on the same form. They chart their observations, plans of action, treatments, and results, with a number telling which particular problem they are working on. The

| LAKESIDE HOSPITAL AND HEALTH CARE CENTER | 7209 347841-6 m 28-447 |
| Patient Record | TIMMONS, RALPH DR. THOMAS MOORE 1-PROT 5/06/20 |

| ALLERGIES Penicillin | BLOOD TYPE AB+ |

PROBLEM NUMBER	DATE	PROBLEM DESCRIPTION	DATE RESOLVED
#1	3/25/94	Diabetes mellitus, insulin-controlled	
#2	3/25/94	Left hand 2nd degree burn	
#3	3/25/94	Wife seriously ill	

Progress Notes

PROBLEM NO. & DESCRIPTION	SUBJECTIVE(S)-OBJECTIVE(O)-ASSESSMENT(A)-PLAN(P)
#2 - LH burn	S: Complains of insomnia, "tossed and turned all night"; LH painful.
	O: Dark circles under eyes, bed sheets rumpled; no change in burn wound appearance.
	A: No pain relief from analgesic. May need larger dose and/or a sedative.
	P: Give backrub. Notify Dr. Moore.
	L. Parker, LPN

Figure 5-22 Problem-oriented medical record (POMR); problem list and progress notes.

list of problems includes any social and psychological factors in the patient's life that may have an effect on treatment. The POMR is designed to make sure that all members of the health care team are aware of what the others are doing and planning for the patient. In this way, the patient receives coordinated care.

Where the POMR is in use, patient progress is often charted by the **SOAP** (subjective–objective–assessment–plan) method. This is a way of organizing the information to be charted. If you wanted to make a note about an unusual reaction to a medication, you would write the information in the order S–O–A–P, as follows:

• Subjective data—the patient's complaints and feelings in his or her own words

• Objective data—your own observations or measurements (e.g., blood pressure, appetite)

• Assessment—what you think may be wrong with the patient

• Plan—treatments, diagnostic tests, medications, or patient education that might help the patient's current problem

Figure 5-22 shows how a health worker might chart the fact that a patient appears to be in pain.

Nursing Home Clinic Charts

In the clinic of a nursing home, the forms used for charting are different from those used on a hospital ward. Usually there is no medication record. Rather, any drugs administered will be charted on a patient history sheet or on the nurses' notes. Again, all of the important information must be charted: drug name, strength and/or amount, route, time of administration, your signature and title, and any other notes about the patient or the drug.

PRINCIPLES OF CHARTING

Because the chart is a record of treatment of a patient, it must record only facts. This means that you must write down only things you did or saw or heard the patient say. Your own conclusions and opinions about a patient's behavior are not to be charted. The only exception to this rule is in the SOAP method of charting, which calls for your assessment of the patient's problem. In this case it is clear that you are giving your own conclusions.

Why are facts better than opinion in charting? Let us take an example. If you found Mrs. Smith in her room crying, you would not write on the chart "depressed about upcoming operation." Instead, you would write "was crying," since there could be many reasons. Suppose that Mr. Jones gagged on a tablet this morning. If you wrote down "doesn't like medicine" on the chart (your opinion of the situation), your information would be misleading. Perhaps there was a physical problem developing that caused Mr. Jones to have trouble swallowing. The chart would show the problem more clearly if you wrote simply "gagged on tablet."

Another important feature of charting is that it is a summary of events. It has to be concise and to the point. There is simply not enough room to record every detail. This is why abbreviations are useful. They allow you to say a great deal in a small amount of space. Learn them well and use them carefully so that others can understand what you have written. It is also useful to learn the proper medical terms for symptoms and body functions. These are understood by most people in the health care field, and they are a kind of shorthand for complicated explanations.

Charting is not difficult, but it requires some practice. Your own charting will be successful if you follow a few simple rules:

- Before you begin, make sure you have the right chart.
- Chart medications directly from a medicine card or a medication record. If neither of these forms is being used, chart directly from the patient chart.
- Chart only after you have given a drug, never before.
- Be specific. Do not write "Gave Demerol for pain in the evening." Instead, write "[date] 2000, Demerol 100 mg I.M. for pain in left arm."
- Write down events in the order in which they occurred.
- Mark D/C for discontinued after the last dose of a drug is given (see Figure 5-11 or 5-12), or cross out the remaining scheduled times, as required by your agency. The doctor will have specified the day and time of the last dose.
- Do not leave gaps or skip lines. If a note does not fill up a complete line, draw a straight line to fill the gap. Put your signature at the right-hand side directly after the note.
- If you make an error, do not erase it. Draw a line through the mistake. It should still be visible; do not black it out! Initial it, and write the word error on the line. Then rechart the information correctly.
- Never use ditto marks in charting.

CONFIDENTIAL REPORT OF INCIDENT (Not part of medical record)

NAME AND ADDRESS OF PERSON INVOLVED. GIVE MEDICAL RECORD NUMBER. USE ADDRESSOGRAPH IF AVAILABLE.	IDENTIFICATION	SEX	AGE	TIME LOST (Employees Only)	NURSES STA. NO.
	☐ 1-Patient ☐ 2-Employee ☐ 3-Visitor	☐ 1-Female ☐ 2-Male		☐ 1-Yes (If unknown, check "No.") ☐ 2-No	
	(19)	(20)	(21-23)	(24)	(25-29)

	INCIDENT DATE	REPORT DATE	INCIDENT		HOSPITAL CODE NOS.
			SHIFT	TIME	STATE (2 Digits) HOSP. NUMBER (3 Digits)
	(Digits Only)	(Digits Only)	☐ 01-1st ☐ 02-2nd ☐ 03-3rd	: ___ A.M. : ___ P.M.	
(1-18)	(30-35)	(36-41)	(42-43)		(44-48)

CONDITION BEFORE	BED ADJUSTMENT	LOCATION OF INCIDENT		NATURE OF INJURY (Injury sustained as a result of incident)
(Patients Only)	(Not Bed Rails)	☐ 400 Admitting	☐ 510 Patients Bathroom	☐ 100 Asphyxia, Strangulation, Inhalation
	(Patients Only)	☐ 410 Offices	☐ 520 Nurses Station	☐ 110 Burn or Scald
1-Normal		☐ 420 Elevators	☐ 530 Surgery and Recovery	☐ 120 Chemical Burn
2-Senile	1-Not Applicable	☐ 430 Corridors	☐ 540 Delivery, Labor & Recovery	☐ 130 Concussion
3-Disoriented		☐ 440 S		
4-Sedated	2-Up	☐ 450 C		
5-Unconscious	3-Down	I		
6-Other		☐ 460 H		
		☐ 470 D		
		☐ 480 L		
		☐ 490 E		
(49)	(50)	☐ 500 P		

INCIDENT CAUSE (57-58) If more than one († Use only for patient incidents.)

A-Falls
☐ 1-Bed, Rail Up
☐ 2-Bed, Rail Down
☐ 3-From Chair or Equip.
☐ 4-From Different Level
☐ 5-On Same Level
☐ 6-Fainting

B-Medication
☐ 7-Patient Iden
☐ 8-Dosage
☐ 9-Route
☐ 10-Unordered
☐ 11-Duplication
☐ 12-Omission

IF PATIENT
Out-Of-Bed Privileges? ☐ Yes ☐ No
Cause for Hospitalization: _____

Room No. _____ Attending Physician: _____

GIVE BRIEF DESCRIPTION OF INCIDENT.
_____
_____
_____
_____

INJURY: _____
PREDOMINANT AND CONTRIBUTING CAUSE
_____
_____

EQUIPMENT INVOLVED: _____

STATE CORRECTIVE ACTION TAKEN, INDI
_____
_____
_____

List all patients in the room. Give names
_____
_____

Was person seen by a physician? ☐ Yes
If Yes , time seen: _____ A.
Name and Address of HOSPITAL

ACCIDENT OR INCIDENT REPORT

(Report all accidents or incidents even if no apparent injury)

Family Name	First Name	Middle Name	Room No.	Bed No.	Admission No.

Date of accident or incident _____ 19___ Time _____ a.m. p.m. Place _____

Was it neccessary to notify physician? yes ___ no ___ Time of notification _____ a.m. p.m.

Name of physician _____ Name of supervising nurse _____

Describe nature of accident or incident and injuries received: _____
_____
_____
_____
_____
_____
_____
_____
_____

Illustrate on the diagram position or place of injury, if any: _____

Date report written _____ 19 ___ Time _____ a.m. p.m. Signed _____

PHYSICIAN OR NURSE

FORM NH-310(X)   PHYSICIANS' RECORD CO., BEDWYN, ILLINOIS · PRINTED IN U.S.A.   ACCIDENT OR INCIDENT REPORT

Figure 5-23   Incident report forms.

- Write with a pen, not a pencil. Only pen will ensure a permanent record. Some agencies require you to use a certain color of ink.
- Always print or write legibly when charting. You may print or you may write neatly in longhand.
- Always use proper abbreviations and symbols when charting. This is very important.
- Chart anything that seems important to you in regard to medication administration.
- Consult the nurse in charge when in doubt about a charting rule.
- The patient chart is to be kept strictly confidential. Do your part to make sure that only authorized people see the chart or discuss its contents. Find out what your agency's policy is and follow it.

Reporting Medication Errors

A medication error is a serious concern. A medication error occurs when you:
- Give a drug to the wrong patient
- Give the wrong medicine
- Give the wrong dose
- Give the drug by the wrong route
- Give the drug at the wrong time

Any of these five situations must be reported immediately to the nurse in charge. The error must be noted in the nurses' notes in the patient chart. An **incident report** or a **medication error form** must also be filled out (Figure 5-23). This form is to be signed by the health worker who made the error and by the nurse in charge. Many health facilities require that the patient be seen by a doctor after the medication error. In this case, the doctor must fill out a section on the form and sign it. The doctor's orders for further patient care must be followed carefully. Remember, telling the truth about an error is better from a legal standpoint than trying to cover it up or make excuses. Not reporting an error at all may seriously harm your patient.

As a final step, review the events that led to the error. Errors may occur for many reasons: copying orders incorrectly, not paying close attention while setting up medications, carrying out procedures automatically without thinking, or failing to communicate with other members of the health care team. Figure out how the error happened and avoid that situation the next time you administer medications.

• • • PRACTICE PROCEDURE 5-1 • • •

Transcribe Medication Orders

Equipment

- Physician's order sheet with at least five drugs ordered
- Kardex and medicine cards or medication record (the forms used by your agency)

Procedure

1. Read the medication orders on the physician's order sheet.
2. Transcribe each order onto the Kardex, if used by your agency. Use proper medical terms and abbreviations. Be sure to record all necessary information, including:

- Name of patient, room number, and bed number.
- Name of drug.
- Route.
- Dosage (strength and frequency of administration).
- Time(s) of administration.
- Special administration or nursing instructions, if any.

3. Transcribe each order onto a medicine card or medication record. Include the same information as in (2).
4. Check off each order as you finish transcribing it onto the medication record or medicine card.
5. Sign or initial the doctor's order after each set of orders is transcribed.

Show your work to your instructor or the nurse in charge.

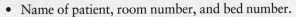

• • • PRACTICE PROCEDURE 5-2 • • •

Write Down Verbal Medication Orders

♦ **NOTE** ♦ ♦ ♦ ♦ ♦ ♦ ♦ ♦ ♦ ♦ ♦ ♦ ♦ ♦ ♦ ♦

Agency policy determines which staff members are allowed to write down doctor's verbal orders.

Equipment

- Oral or tape-recorded statements of at least five medication orders
- Physician's order sheet (in a patient chart) or doctor's order book

Procedure

1. Listen closely to the verbal medication orders.
2. Record the orders on the physician's order sheet or order book. Be sure to:
   - Include all the necessary information (patient's name, date, drug name, dosage, route).
   - Use proper medical terms and abbreviations.
   - Skip a line between orders.
   - Write neatly with a ballpoint pen.
3. Read the orders back to the physician (or the instructor) afterward.
4. Record the physician's name and then your name. State how you received the orders, in person or by phone (e.g., "Dr. E.S. MacLean/phone order taken by P.T. Bayt)". Remember that for the order to be legal, the physician will have to sign it personally as soon as possible.

Show your work to your instructor or the nurse in charge.

Count Controlled Substances

◆ **NOTE** ◆ ◆ ◆ ◆ ◆ ◆ ◆ ◆ ◆ ◆ ◆ ◆ ◆ ◆ ◆ ◆ ◆

In a laboratory setting, this procedure should be practiced with a partner. Pretend that one of you is going off duty and the other is coming on duty.

Equipment

- Controlled substance folder with the forms used by your agency (sign-in/out form, proof-of-use records for several drugs)
- Locked box, cabinet, or drawer and keys
- Sample containers of controlled substances (divided containers, multiple-dose bottles (tablet or capsules and liquids), unit-dose packages, etc.)

Procedure

1. The person coming on duty obtains the key to the controlled-substance storage area from the person going off duty. Some areas have double doors and require two keys.

2. Unlock the controlled-substance cabinet, box, or drawer in the medicine room. Remove the containers.

3. Count the amount of medicine in each container.
   - *Divided containers (tablets or capsules).* Look for the slot that has the last tablet or capsule in it. The number of this slot is the number of tablets left.
   - *Unit-dose packages.* Unit doses will be numbered. The package with the highest number tells how many doses are left.
   - *Multiple-dose bottles (tablets or capsules).* Tip the bottle on its side and count the contents.
   - *Multiple-dose bottles (liquids).* The bottle should be marked off in cubic centimeters or milliliters. Hold the bottle at eye level and note how many cubic centimeters or milliliters are left.

4. As you finish counting each drug, write the quantity on the appropriate form. Each drug will have a form to go with it. If the form is a proof-of-use record, check that your count matches the amount of drug shown as still available. Different facilities will have different ways to do this. Sign your name where requested.

5. If your count differs from the number shown in the records, do a recount. If there is still a difference, look at the Kardex and other forms to locate the source of error. Notify the nurse in charge if the source of error cannot be found.

6. Correct errors on your forms according to the policy of your health facility.

7. Sign any of the forms required by your agency (sign-in/out, key count, etc.).

8. Return medications to the lock-box and close and lock the doors. Return the controlled-substance folder to the place where it is kept.

9. The person who has just come on duty keeps the key(s) for use in administering controlled substances during the next shift.

Show your work to your instructor or the nurse in charge.

• • • PRACTICE PROCEDURE 5-4 • • •

Record the Use of Controlled Substances

Equipment

- Locked storage area (box, cabinet, or drawer) and keys
- Medication record, medicine cards, or Kardex with several orders for controlled substances
- Proof-of-use records for several controlled substances
- Sample containers of controlled substances (unit dose, multiple dose)

Procedure

1. Unlock storage area and read medication orders. Follow Steps 2 through 7 for one medication at a time.
2. Read the label as you remove a container from the storage area.
3. Pick out the proof-of-use form that goes with that drug. Fill out the form, giving the date of administration, time of administration, patient's full name, room and bed number, amount of medication taken from the container, patient's physician, name of the person giving the medication, and the amount of medication given to the patient.
4. Get someone to act as a witness if you have to discard some of the medication. You may have to discard medication if:
   - You must give a smaller amount than the smallest unit-dose size.
   - You suspect that a drug is contaminated.

   The witness should sign the proof-of-use record and state how much of the drug was destroyed.
5. Set up the medication as you would any other. Be sure to read the label again as you open the container.
6. Replace the container in the storage area. Read the label one last time as you do so.
7. Repeat these steps for the remaining controlled substances.
8. Lock the storage area and replace the controlled-substance folder. Keep the keys in your pocket for use on duty.

Show your work to your instructor or the nurse in charge.

• • • PRACTICE PROCEDURE 5-5 • • •

Set Up Medications on a Tray With Medicine Cards

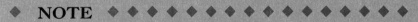

> ◆ **NOTE** ◆ ◆ ◆ ◆ ◆ ◆ ◆ ◆ ◆ ◆ ◆ ◆ ◆ ◆ ◆
>
> This same procedure may be used to set up a medicine cart when you have multiple-dose packages. If the drawers of the cart are marked with patients' names, you may set up from a medication record rather than from medicine cards.

Equipment

- Medicine cards
- Medicine tray (either flat or molded)

- Containers of medicine (unit dose and multiple dose)
- Paper cups for tablets or capsules, plastic cups for liquids
- Supplies (water and water cups, tongue blades, spoons, blood pressure cuff, applesauce or juice for mixing medications, if necessary)

Procedure

1. Set up one medication at a time. Place one card on the tray. You need the medicine card to be able to tell which medicine goes to which patient.

2. Read the label as you take the appropriate medicine container from the cabinet, refrigerator, or medicine cart. Hold the label at eye level.

3. Before opening the container, check the label against the medicine card.

4. Pour or count out the drug into plastic or paper cups. Double-check the dose against the medicine card after you have poured or counted out the medication.

5. Set the medicine cup on the tray next to its medicine card. By setting up only one drug at a time, you make sure that you will put the right card with the right medication. (Refer back to Figure 5-8 to see how a typical tray is set up.)

6. Measure liquids at eye level. Pour with the label away from the side on which you are pouring.

7. Read the label again as you put away the container. Be sure to wipe off any spilled medication.

8. Place any needed supplies on the tray for administering the medications.

9. Follow Steps 1 through 8 as you set up the remaining medications, one at a time.

Show your work to your instructor or the nurse in charge.

• • • PRACTICE PROCEDURE 5-6 • • •

Dispense Unit-Dose Medications From a Cart

Equipment

- Folder with medication records
- Medicine cart, drawers labeled with names of patients
- Unit doses of medicine placed in appropriate drawers of medicine cart
- Medicine cart supplies (water, cups, spoons, etc.)

Procedure

1. Open folder to first patient's medication record.

2. Go to that patient's room and identify the patient by:
   - Checking the name on the wristband or on the bed.
   - Asking the patient his or her name.
   - Asking personnel to help you identify any patient who seems confused or who does not have a wristband or a bed tag.

3. Open the appropriate patient's drawer, identify the right medication, and give it to the patient, following these steps:
   - Read the medication record and identify the medication.
   - Read the label of the unit-dose package and compare it with the medication record.
   - Read the label of the unit-dose package as you give it to the patient.
   - Read the label of the unit-dose package as you discard it.

4. Chart administration of each drug on the medication record.

5. Make the patient comfortable.

6. Go to the next patient's room. This should be the patient whose medication record is next in the medication folder.

Show your work to your instructor or the nurse in charge.

• • • PRACTICE PROCEDURE 5-7 • • •

Fill Out an Incident Report Form

▶ **Equipment**

- Incident report form (the form that is used by your agency)
- Written or oral summary of an actual or made-up medication error (a tape recording or a written story)

▶ **Procedure**

1. Read or listen to the report of a medication error.
2. Record all information requested on the appropriate incident/accident form. Usually this includes:
   - Name, room number, and bed of the patient.
   - Date, time, and location of the incident.
   - Name of the doctor or supervisor who was notified of the incident.
   - Nature of the incident or accident and injuries received.
   - Diagram of the location of the injury on the body.
   - Date and time of this report.
   - Your signature.
3. Obtain signatures of all persons involved as required on the form.

Show your work to your instructor or the nurse in charge.

CHAPTER 5 REVIEW

Using Medical Terminology

Match the medical forms to their descriptions.

_____ 1. Medications ordered by the physician in a hospital

_____ 2. Details of the development and symptoms of a patient's disease

_____ 3. Observations of the patient, nursing care, and stat and PRN medications

_____ 4. Form for charting medications administered on a regular schedule

_____ 5. One form used to chart care given by all health team members

_____ 6. Doctor's orders for an outpatient

_____ 7. Signed after administering narcotics

_____ 8. Placed next to each dose of medication on a medicine tray

a. POMR
b. proof-of-use record
c. medicine card
d. nurses' notes
e. doctor's order sheet
f. patient history sheet
g. prescription blank
h. incident report form
i. Kardex file
j. medication record

_____ 9. Summary of daily medications and treatments for all patients on the ward

_____ 10. Used to record medication errors

Acquiring Knowledge of Medications

Answer the following questions in the spaces provided.

11. List two forms that can be used to order drugs from the pharmacy. _____

_____

12. How many doses of medication are contained in a unit-dose package? _____

_____

13. How many doses of medication are contained in a multiple-dose package? _____

_____

14. What must be counted or measured at the beginning of each shift? _____

_____

15. List two examples of controlled substances. _____

_____

16. Where should controlled substances be stored? _____

_____

17. List two types of drugs that often require refrigeration. _____

_____

18. Why must a medicine room be kept clean at all times? _____

_____

19. Why do some drugs have to be stored in a dark place? _____

_____

20. How will you know if a particular drug needs to be refrigerated? _____

_____

21. What should you do with unused doses from a stock supply bottle? _____

_____

22. List two advantages of single-dose packaging. _____

_____

_____

23. Where should drugs labeled "for external use only" be kept? _____

_____

24. How do you know if a medication is usable? _____

_____

25. How can you tell if a medication has been stored improperly? _____
_____

26. How can you best make a clean break when dividing a scored tablet? _____
_____

27. List the five rights of medication administration. _____
_____
_____
_____
_____
_____

28. What should you do on the medication record after giving the last dose of a medication? _____
_____

29. When administering drugs in a clinic or office, where do you chart them? _____
_____

30. List two rules for administering medications. _____
_____
_____

31. List two rules for giving the correct medication. _____
_____
_____

32. List two rules for giving the proper dose of a medication. _____
_____
_____

33. List two rules for using the appropriate route. _____
_____
_____

34. List three rules for giving the patient's medicine at the right time. _____
_____
_____
_____

35. List three reasons why the patient chart is an important document. _____
_____
_____
_____

36. What six types of information must be charted whenever a medication is given? _____

_____

_____

_____

37. List the three times you should read the label as you prepare a medication for your patient. _____

_____

38. What is the SOAP system of charting? _____

_____

_____

39. On a medication record, how would you show that a dose of medicine was not given when scheduled? (Check the procedure in your own agency.)

_____

_____

_____

40. How would you show that a dose of medicine was given? (Check the procedure in your own agency.)

_____

_____

Applying Knowledge on the Job

Show how you would chart the following events in the nurses' notes. Be sure to include all of the required information. Remember that only facts are to be charted, not assumptions or opinions.

Mr. Schwartz is under treatment for a blood clot in the leg. He has been taking *Coumadin*, an anticoagulant, for several days. He is also taking *Diuril*, a diuretic, to reduce the swelling in his leg. The doctor has confined Mr. Schwartz to bed. This is because any movement of the leg might cause the clot to break off and travel in the bloodstream, which could be dangerous.

41. At 0800 on October 5, 1994, you give Mr. Schwartz two 5-mg tablets of *Coumadin* to swallow with a glass of water. You chart it on the medication record. As you refill the water pitcher, Mr. Schwartz asks if you happen to have something for an upset stomach. He says his stomach hurts the way it did when he had an ulcer 20 years ago. Because the anticoagulant can cause internal bleeding (e.g., from an old ulcer), you have been alert for signs of this side effect. You notify your supervisor, who asks the doctor to order a test for internal bleeding. The test results are negative. The supervisor then directs you to give Mr. Schwartz 2 tsp of *Maalox* to calm his stomach.

_____

_____

_____

42. It is 1200 hours and time for Mr. Schwartz's next dose of *Diuril*. Mr. Schwartz complains again about his upset stomach, but this time he tells you it is worse right after he takes the *Diuril*. You skip this dose of *Diuril* and notify the supervisor. The supervisor tells you to continue giving the *Diuril* but to keep an eye out for signs of internal bleeding.

_____

_____

_____
_____
_____

43. It is 2000 hours the next evening and time to give Mr. Schwartz a laxative. The laxative *(Dulcolax)* has been ordered by the doctor because bedridden patients often develop constipation, which can lead to impaction (blocking of the intestine). Straining during a bowel movement might cause the blood clot to break off and become an embolism (a traveling clot). Mr. Schwartz tells you that he has been having regular bowel movements and doesn't want the laxative. He asks why he needs it when he has been in bed for only 2 days. You explain that it is preventive medicine to avoid the problems of impaction and embolism. But Mr. Schwartz doesn't seem to listen to your explanation. He seems nervous about his condition. He refuses the laxative. You then notify the supervisor. After consulting with the doctor, the supervisor instructs you to give Mr. Schwartz 10 mg of *Valium* intramuscularly right away. *Valium* is a tranquilizer that will ease Mr. Schwartz's anxiety so that he can cooperate with the treatment.

_____
_____
_____
_____
_____
_____
_____

Using Resources on the Job

Obtain a current copy of the PDR from your school, nursing unit, or clinic. Use it to answer the questions that follow.

44. What is the name of the section where the listing of unit-dose systems is given? _____

_____

45. In this section, locate the drug spironolactone *(Aldactone)*. How is this drug supplied as a unit dose? _____

_____
_____

46. In the same section, locate diazepam *(Valium)*. What information does the manufacturer give about unit-dose systems?

_____

→ ANSWERS TO CHAPTER 5 REVIEW ←

Using Medical Terminology

1. e	2. f	3. d
4. j	5. a	6. g
7. b	8. c	9. i
10. h		

Acquiring Knowledge of Medications

11. Doctor's order sheet, pharmacy requisition

12. One

13. More than one

14. Controlled substances

15. Narcotics, barbiturates, amphetamines, hallucinogens, etc.

16. In a locked cabinet

17. Vaccines, eyedrops, suppositories

18. To avoid medication errors

19. Because light causes a chemical breakdown

20. The drug label will say so.

21. Dispose of them according to agency policy.

22. There is less chance of error because no mixing, pouring, or handling of drugs is needed. Unused doses can be returned to the pharmacy for credit.

23. In a labeled cabinet separate from the drugs for internal use.

24. Check the expiration date on the label.

25. You may notice a change in the color, odor, or texture.

26. Use a knife edge.

27. Right patient, right drug, right dose, right time, right route

28. Write D/C (discontinued).

29. Patient history sheet

30. Check the patient's wrist identification band. Ask the nurse in charge to help identify the patient. Ask the patient his or her name—unless the patient is groggy or confused.

31. Give medicine from labeled containers. Read the label three times.

32. Use properly marked measuring containers. Know dosage measurements and abbreviations.

33. Be aware of changes or factors in the patient's condition that may affect the route. Know the abbreviations for routes.

34. Organize your time or workday. Know the abbreviations for administration times. Check to see if the medication should be given on a full or empty stomach.

35. It serves as a means of communication among members of the health care team. It is a legal document, an official record of health care given. It is used for research, teaching, and evaluation of health facilities.

36. Drug names, strength and/or amount of drug, time of administration, route, anything else that seems important about the patient or administration, and signature or initials of the health care worker.

37. While taking it from the storage area, just before opening it, and when putting it away.

38. Charting <u>S</u>ubjective comments of the patient, <u>Ob</u>jective tests of the patient's condition, the health care worker's <u>A</u>ssessment of the problem, and a <u>P</u>lan of action.

39. This depends on the agency. One way is to circle the scheduled time and initial it.

40. This depends on the agency. One way is to cross out the scheduled time and initial it.

Applying Knowledge on the Job

41. 10/5/94 0800 — Complained of abdominal pain & requested med. for upset stomach. Stated pain is like ulcer pain experienced previously. Supervisor notified. Hematcrit ordered. — negative. Maalox 2T given as ordered. Your name, Title

42. 10/5/94 1200 — Said stomach pain most severe after taking Dinril. Withheld Dinril & notified supervisor. Orders given to continue Dinril and observe for bleeding ——— Your name, Title

43. 10/6/94 2000 — Refused Ducolax. Possible complications such as impaction & embolism explained. Notified supervisor. Valium 10 mg IM given stat for agitation. ——— Your name, Title

Using Resources on the Job

44. At the end of Section 3, Product Category Index.

45. 25-mg tablets, 50-mg tablets, 100-mg tablets

46. Available in 2-mg, 5-mg, or 10-mg tablets and as a prefilled, disposable 2-ml syringe.

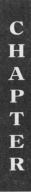
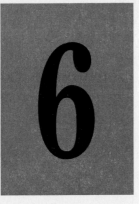

C H A P T E R

6 Drugs for Infection and Cancer

◆◆ In this chapter you will learn basic facts about cells, tissues, organs, and systems. This is your introduction to the study of specific body systems in later units. You will then learn about two types of disorders that can affect any system of the body: infection and cancer. You will learn how these disorders affect the body and how drugs are used to treat them. You will also learn how health care workers can stop the spread of germs.

COMPETENCIES

After studying this chapter, you should be able to

- use proper terms for discussing cells, tissues, organs, and body systems.
- name the four types of body cells.
- list substances that the body must take in.
- differentiate between the external and internal immune systems.
- explain why infection is more dangerous in a hospital or long-term care unit than elsewhere.
- state the two main actions of anti-infectives on germs.
- explain why drug resistance, drug sensitivity, and superinfection are important concerns in anti-infective drug therapy.
- name at least two problems that may arise in giving penicillin.
- list the most common uses of sulfonamides and gamma globulin.
- name the three characteristics of all cancers.
- explain how chemotherapy works.
- list the signs to look for when working with patients on chemotherapy.
- name at least three groups of antineoplastic drugs and give examples.
- describe the correct procedure for washing your hands before and after giving medications.
- state three primary ways a health care worker can be exposed to hepatitis B virus and human immunodeficiency virus.
- explain the universal blood and body fluid precautions.

AIDS: acquired immune deficiency syndrome

anaphylaxis: severe, possibly fatal systemic hypersensitivity reaction to a sensitizing agent, that is, a drug, food, or chemical

antibiotic: substance produced by a living microorganism that kills or stops the growth of other organisms (can also be produced in the laboratory)

antibody: a proteinlike substance produced in the body to fight germs

anti-infective: drug that kills germs or keeps them from growing

antineoplastic: drug that suppresses cancer cells and other growing cells

aseptic: free of pathogens

autoclave: sterilizing machine

bactericidal: destructive to bacteria

bacteriostatic: an agent that inhibits the growth or multiplication of bacteria

benign: harmless; unable to spread to other parts of the body

biocidal activity: the ability to kill microorganisms

biostatic activity: the ability to inhibit the growth of a microorganism

biotechnology: biogenetic engineering; the ability to make proteins that are normally produced in the body

broad spectrum: affecting a wide variety of pathogens

cell: the basic unit of structure of all living things

chemotherapy: drug therapy for cancer symptoms (also refers to drug therapy of other types)

culture and sensitivity test: laboratory technique for finding out which microbes are present, if any, and which anti-infective will be effective against a specific pathogen

cytoplasm: fluid inside the cells

cytostatic: able to suppress cell growth and replication

cytotoxic: poisonous to cells

disinfectant: substance for sterilizing tools and equipment

extravasation: discharge of blood or other substances into tissues

gamma globulin: a class of protein in the bloodstream that includes antibodies

Gram stain: laboratory test to help identify microbes

HBV: hepatitis B virus

HIV: human immunodeficiency virus

hypersensitivity: an exaggerated response to a drug or other foreign agent through allergic mechanisms

immunity: the body's ability to resist many pathogens

immunization: a way of stimulating production of antibodies by exposing the body to weakened or killed germs

infection: an invasion by pathogens that causes symptoms

infectious disease: disease caused by the direct or indirect spread of pathogens from one person to another

inoculation: immunizing by administration of a vaccine

isolation: keeping a patient in an environment where pathogens cannot spread from patient to health care worker and/or vice versa

leukocytes: white blood cells that destroy germ cells

leukopenia: reduction in the number of the leukocytes in the blood, that is, 4000 or less

macrolide: another name for erythromycin

malignant: cancerous; able to spread to other parts of the body or to invade locally

metastasis: spread of a cancer by "seeding" cancer cells to other parts of the body

microbes: another name for microorganisms

microorganisms: tiny, one-celled plants and animals; some are beneficial to humans, and others are harmful; also called microbes

narrow spectrum: affecting only specific pathogens

organ: two or more tissue types that perform a specific function

pathogens: harmful microorganisms

penicillinase: enzyme produced by microbes that makes them resistant to penicillin

photosensitivity: rash that appears after exposure to strong light; a side effect of some drugs

remission: disappearance of disease symptoms

resistance: a germ's developed ability to withstand drug effects after a period of drug therapy

sulfonamide: a type of synthetic anti-infective; sulfa

superinfection: second infection that starts while an antibiotic is destroying the first infection

system: group of organs that carry out one set of important life processes (e.g., eating, breathing, elimination)

tissue: group of cells of the same type, working together to perform some function

tissue fluid: fluid found in spaces between cells; also called intercellular fluid

tumor: abnormal lump or mass of tissue

vaccination: immunizing by introducing into the body dead or weakened viruses, either orally or by skin puncture

INTRODUCTION TO BODY SYSTEMS

The human body is a marvelously complex machine. In Chapter 2 you learned something about how it responds to the actions of drugs. Beginning with this chapter, you will learn about the various parts of the body and their structure and function. Your knowledge of how different parts of the body work will help you in administering medications. You will understand what goes wrong with body parts during disease or malfunction. You will also understand why doctors prescribe specific drugs for each condition. Armed with this knowledge, you will be a more responsible member of the health care team.

Cells

Cells are the basic unit of structure of all living things. There are millions of them in every human body. Each cell carries out certain routine functions to keep itself alive—absorbing food; creating energy for heat, growth, or movement; excreting waste products; and reproducing itself when conditions are right. But each cell works with other cells, too, to carry out more complex activities that keep the whole body working smoothly.

For efficiency, cells are specialized to do certain jobs. Some are designed to form protective coatings and linings for body parts. Some specialize in producing chemicals that control body processes. Others are specialized for connecting body parts or creating body movement. Still others have the job of sending messages to and from the body's main control center, the brain.

There are four types of cells in the human body, each with its own special job: epithelial cells, connective cells, muscle cells, and nerve cells (Figure 6-1).

Cells have the ability to split in two when they have reached a certain size. This is called cell reproduction. The two cells that result from this division are exactly alike. They will do the same job in the body as the original cell. Cell

Epithelial cells
Linings of body tubes and cavities
Glands
Skin

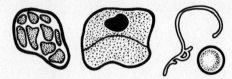

Connective cells
Bones, ligaments, cartilage
Scar tissue

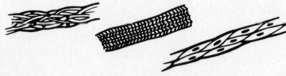

Muscle cells
Muscles that move bones
Smooth muscles in internal organs
Heart muscle

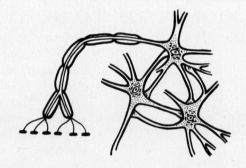

Nerve cells
Brain
Spinal cord
Sense receptors
Nerves

Figure 6-1 The four types of cells, with some of the body parts they make up.

reproduction enables living things to grow. As cells divide and redivide, the body grows larger. At some point this process stops: the human body reaches its full adult size. From then on, cells reproduce themselves only to replace worn-out or damaged cells.

During disease and trauma, many cells may be damaged. But because cells can reproduce themselves, the body can often replace the damaged cells. This is called healing.

As the body grows older, the process of cell division begins to slow down. Cells are not able to replace themselves as easily as they did in youth. Consequently, the body takes a longer time to heal after an accident or an illness. The routine processes of digesting, producing energy, and excreting waste all slow down, too. This is why older people have special medical needs and why drug doses have to be adjusted for age.

Tissues, Organs, and Systems

Cells are specialized to do certain jobs, but they do not do these jobs alone. They work together with other cells that have the same specialty. These groups of cells that together perform a certain function are called **tissues.**

Four basic types of tissues, corresponding to the four types of cells, make up all of the body parts: epithelial tissue, connective tissue, muscle tissue, and nerve tissue. Each type of tissue has a different structure and function.

After cells and tissues, organs are the next most complex structures in the human body. Organs are made up of two or more types of tissues, organized to carry out a particular function. The heart, the liver, the stomach, and the kidneys are familiar examples of organs. Some people consider skin and blood to be organs, too.

The important functions that keep the body alive—breathing, eating and digesting, elimination, thinking, and regulating the body processes—are performed by well-organized groups of organs and tissues called body **systems.** Each system is responsible for one important body function.

There are 10 major systems in the human body. You will learn more about these systems as you study the remaining chapters of this text. You will learn what their parts are; how they function; and what can go wrong with them when they are injured, diseased, or aged. This will give you a better understanding of how they are affected by drugs and why specific drugs are given.

NECESSARY SUBSTANCES

The body is built of living cells, and it can make many substances that it needs. However, there are some materials that the body must take in.

Water is the most important of these substances. In fact, about 66% of the body is composed of water. Water is the largest component of the fluid inside cells, or **cytoplasm.**

Water also surrounds the cells, bathing every tissue in fluid. This is important because water is the medium through which most of the body's chemical activities take place. Gases, liquids, and solids are dissolved in water before traveling through the body. The processes of absorption, distribution, biotransformation, and excretion all involve water. The water that surrounds the cells is known as **tissue fluid.**

Other substances that the body depends on for its life processes are minerals such as salt (tissue fluid is slightly salty) and calcium (for the hardness in bones and teeth), vitamins, fats, carbohydrates, and proteins. A well-balanced diet ensures that the body takes in a good supply of these necessary substances.

INFECTION AND IMMUNITY

We are literally surrounded by tiny, one-celled plants and animals—called germs or, more properly, **microorganisms** or **microbes.** They are in the air we breathe, on the food we eat, and on the things we touch. Many of them are harmless. Some are even beneficial; for example, certain bacteria that live in the intestine help create important vitamins out of the waste products of digestion. But some are able to produce infection and disease in the human body. These harmful germs—known as **pathogens**—are responsible for everything from the common cold to malaria, Colorado tick fever, and spinal meningitis (Figure 6-2).

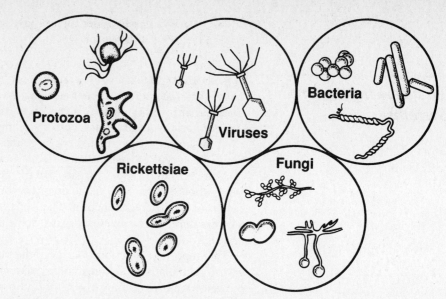

Figure 6-2 These pathogens can cause infection.

When they get a foothold in the body, they reproduce rapidly and start to affect healthy tissue, causing symptoms.

Infectious diseases have distinct sets of symptoms that help in diagnosis. Fever, chills, headache, nausea, vomiting, diarrhea, and pus formation at the infection site are some of the signs that a physician takes into consideration. Laboratory tests confirm the diagnosis by identifying the specific germ that caused the disease. Identifying the germ is very important because different drugs are effective against different types of germs. Table 6-1 lists the major types of infectious diseases.

TABLE 6-1: Infectious Diseases

Bacterial Infections
  Anthrax
  Bacillary dysentery
  Bacterial endocarditis
  Blood poisoning
  Boils
  Botulism
  Brucellosis (undulant fever)
  Cholera
  Diphtheria
  Gastroenteritis (food poisoning)
  Gonorrhea
  Meningitis
  Osteomyelitis
  Plague
  Pneumonia
  Strep throat
  Tetanus
  Trench mouth
  Tularemia
  Typhoid fever

Chlamydial Infections

Fungus Infections (mycoses)
  Actinomycosis
  Candidiasis (moniliasis)
  Coccidioidomycosis
  Histoplasmosis

Parasitic Infections
  Flukes
  Hookworm
  Pinworm
  Roundworm
  Schistosomiasis
  Tapeworm
  Trichinosis

Protozoan Infections
  Amebic dysentery (amebiasis)
  Malaria
  Toxoplasmosis
  Trypanosomiasis (sleeping sickness)

Rickettsial Infections
  Rocky Mountain spotted fever
  Typhus

Spirochetal Infections
  Lyme disease
  Syphilis

Virus Infections
  AIDS
  Chickenpox
  Cold sores (herpes simplex)
  Common cold
  Encephalitis
  Genital herpes
  Influenza (flu, grippe)
  Lymphogranuloma
  Measles
  Mononucleosis
  Mumps
  Poliomyelitis
  Psittacosis (parrot fever)
  Rabies
  Shingles (herpes zoster)
  Viral hepatitis
  Yellow fever

The Immune System

The immune system has two parts: external and internal.

External. The external immune system gives protection from infection because of normal functioning defenses. The most important of these is the skin. It provides a tough physical barrier to the entry of germs. When the skin barrier is damaged, such as when cut or burned, many germs can enter the body and cause infection.

Internal. The internal immune system is made up of microscopic substances whose specialized function is to fight infection.

Certain cells, called neutrophils, surround and digest the germ cells. Leukocytes, also called white blood cells, produce antibodies, which are proteins that help destroy germ cells as they enter the body.

Antibodies. Antibodies are proteins that either destroy or stop the growth of certain types of germs. Antibodies are carried in the bloodstream and can readily move to the site of entry.

Specific antibodies act against specific germs. When an unfamiliar germ enters the body, proteins in the blood are stimulated to produce a special antibody to act against it. The next time that same germ enters the body, the antibody "remembers" it and proceeds to destroy it. Antibodies make the body immune to a great many infections.

Immunity can be either temporary or permanent, depending on the type of antibody. People who, for some reason, cannot form antibodies are at risk because they cannot defend themselves against the germs to which we are all constantly exposed.

Despite all of these defenses, germs sometimes get the better of us. They multiply and spread in the body, and the result is infection. The infection can be local, such as in a cut or a surgical wound, or it can be systemic and affect the whole body, as in measles.

Immunization

Because of the pioneering work of Edward Jenner, Jonas Salk, and others, today we are able to prevent many deadly or debilitating infectious diseases that in the past affected many lives. Through **immunization,** we are able to stimulate the body to produce antibodies against the dreaded disease germs. This is done by placing a small amount of dead or weak disease germs into the body, called **inoculation** or **vaccination.** Because the germs are not at full strength, they do not cause a full-blown disease, but they provide enough material so that the body can manufacture the necessary antibodies. Thus, when living germs come along, the antibodies are already there to fight them off. Immunization has been so successful that diseases that used to kill thousands of people during sweeping epidemics, such as measles and yellow fever, are now rare.

Patients at Risk

Most individuals can fight off infection successfully. If they are in good health, their natural defenses hold down the number of germs, so that there are few disease symptoms. Even if the diseases do take hold, healthy people are able to survive while the infection runs its course. It is the people who are *not* healthy who are at risk.

Patients with surgical wounds or with lowered resistance because of other conditions, such as **AIDS** (acquired immune deficiency syndrome), are especially prone to infections. Weak patients are apt to have more serious disease symptoms. They also have a harder time shaking off infections and avoiding complications. Very young and very old people also have less resistance to infection.

Hospitals and other health care facilities have large numbers of these at-risk patients located in one place. Once started, an infection can spread very rapidly through such groups. For this reason, medical personnel must be especially concerned with avoiding the spread of pathogens. They are trained in **aseptic** or

TABLE 6-2: Drug Categories for Infection and Cancer

Antibacterials and Antiseptics	Antibiotics	Antineoplastics
Acne preparations	Amebicides	Analgesics
Antibacterials	Anti-inflammatory agents	Androgen inhibitors
Astringents	Broad- and medium-spectrum	Antibiotic derivatives
Burn relief	Cephalosporins	Antiestrogen
Dandruff medications	Fungal medications	Antimetabolites
Dermatitis relief	Keratolytics	Cytotoxic agents
Fungicides	Monobactams	Hormones
Nail fungus treatment	Penicillin	Nitrogen mustard derivatives
Pediculicides	Tuberculosis	Steroids and combinations
Pruritus	Viral agents	
Parenteral medications	Topicals	
Quinolones		
Sulfonamides		
Sulfonamide combinations		
Topicals		

germ-free techniques of caring for patients. They learn to wash their hands before and after caring for each patient. They learn to sterilize equipment, change bed linens frequently, and wear protective clothing when handling certain infected patients.

There are pathogens that seem to lurk in hospitals waiting to attack weakened patients. Each hospital has its own problem infections caused by antibiotic-resistant germs that gain a foothold in the building. Staph (staphylococcal) infections are a common danger for hospitalized patients. People who develop such infections must be kept in **isolation.** No one may enter or leave these patients' rooms without special precautions against spreading staph germs. Practice Procedure 6-1 at the end of this chapter will show you how to prepare to administer medications to an isolation patient.

ANTI-INFECTIVE DRUGS

The discovery of so-called miracle drugs—the antibiotics—changed the practice of medicine radically. Antibiotics are drugs that destroy microorganisms. There are many different kinds of antimicrobials (see Table 6-2). Many antibiotics are now synthesized as well.

How do these drugs work? Anti-infectives either kill germs directly (indicated by the suffix -*cide*, as in *fungicide*) or keep them from growing (suffix = *static*, as in *bacteriostatic*). Some interfere with cell wall production in the germs. Others inhibit protein synthesis. Still others mix up the chemical messages for producing nucleic acid, a major substance in cell growth. Some act better on rapidly multiplying pathogens, whereas others are more effective with slowly growing organisms.

Administration Considerations

Before prescribing antibiotics for specific ailments, a physician must consider three things:

- *The condition of the patient's own defense system.* The physician must note whether the patient's immune system is working properly. Some antibiotics kill germs directly and others slow the growth or reproduction of germs. Both types depend on the body's natural defenses (leukocytes and antibodies) for help in eliminating an infection.

- *The type of infection and its cause.* The organism causing the infection is important. Some infectious diseases have distinct symptoms, but many have similar symptoms. When in doubt, an attempt must be made to identify the germ. The identity of the pathogen determines the choice of a specific antibiotic. That choice often depends on how the germ behaves in a laboratory test called a **Gram stain.**

  When placed on a microscope slide along with a stain, some microbes turn blue and others turn red. The blue-staining germs are called gram-positive microbes and the red-staining ones gram-negative. The shape of the microbes also may change. These changes, along with the color changes, help identify the right antibiotic to be used. For example, vancomycin is effective against most gram-positive microbes, and tobramycin is effective against most gram-negative microbes.

- *The type of drug and its effects.* The physician must consider the type of antibiotic because these drugs have varying effectiveness and varying side effects. Another laboratory procedure called a **culture and sensitivity test** helps in deciding which drug to use. A sample of fluid (e.g., pus obtained from a throat scraping) is taken from an infected person's body and used to start a culture of bacteria in the laboratory. Then pieces of paper saturated with samples of different anti-infectives are placed on the culture. The results show which drug can kill the bacteria, and this is the drug the doctor will prescribe.

Sometimes it is hard to isolate the germ that is causing an ailment. In these situations a physician might prescribe a **broad-spectrum** antibiotic. This is an antibiotic that destroys a great variety of microorganisms. The cephalosporins are one group of broad-spectrum antibiotics. In contrast, **narrow-spectrum** antibiotics are effective against only a few types of pathogens (Figure 6-3).

Resistance. If the disease-producing organism can be identified, a narrow-spectrum drug is usually a better choice than a broad-spectrum drug. This is because pathogens are able to develop **resistance** to antibiotics. After being exposed to a certain antibiotic for a while, a particular pathogen may no longer be sensitive to its action.

Once this happens, it is useless to continue giving that antibiotic to the patient. (But note that the *germ*, not the *person*, becomes resistant to an antibiotic.) Use of broad-spectrum antibiotics gives more types of organisms a chance to develop resistance. Because of resistance, the overuse of antibiotics is now recognized as an

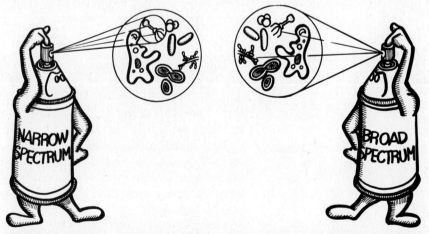

Figure 6-3 Two types of anti-infectives. When a pathogen can be identified, a narrow-spectrum anti-infective is better.

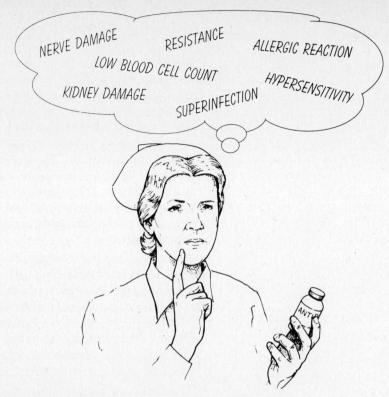

Figure 6-4 Dangers to watch for in administering antibiotics.

important public health problem. The results are seen in hospitals where certain strains of resistant bacteria have appeared, causing hospital-acquired infections.

Sensitivity. Another problem the doctor considers in prescribing anti-infectives is drug **hypersensitivity**. After a few doses of some antibiotics, certain patients become especially sensitive to the drugs and show allergiclike reactions. The doctor must then switch them to another drug that kills the same germs but perhaps has more side effects.

Antibiotics have some serious side effects (see Figure 6-4). Some antibiotics are especially toxic to the kidneys and are thus dangerous for people with kidney problems. The physician weighs the benefits of the drug against the dangers of not giving the drug. Usually the physician has several drugs to choose among, some more dangerous than others. A more dangerous drug is chosen only when a less dangerous one has failed to stop an infection or when the patient has become hypersensitive or resistant to it.

Schedules

Timing is also important. It takes time to wipe out infection, and pathogens may be present long after symptoms are gone. The physician must order the anti-infective for the proper length of time, and those who give medications must see that all doses are taken. This is an important teaching point for patients who will be taking these drugs on their own.

Time of day is also important because doses of anti-infectives must be scheduled with mealtimes in mind. Oral anti-infectives can cause gastric irritation. Giving them on a full stomach or with milk can help soothe the irritation. However, some are made less effective when food or milk is present in the stomach. It is important to find out if oral anti-infectives should be given with food or milk or on an empty stomach. Instructions to "give between meals" mean that the drug is to be given at least 1 hour before or 2 hours after meals, when the stomach is assumed to be empty.

Antibiotics

An antibiotic is a substance with the ability to destroy life. It is produced by a microorganism and has **bactericidal** activity or **bacteriostatic** activity on other microorganisms.

Penicillins. The penicillins are a large group of anti-infective drugs. They come in many forms, to be given by different routes according to the therapeutic aim. Natural penicillins are made from a mold that grows on bread and fruit. Penicillin G potassium *(Pentids)* and penicillin V *(Pen-Vee, V-Cillin K)* are the most common natural penicillins. They are commonly used to treat syphilis and strep throat. Amoxicillin, a type of penicillin, may be given to ward off infections in patients with heart disease and rheumatic fever.

Unfortunately, there are some germs (especially staphylococci, the deadly staph germs) that fight back when attacked by penicillin. They secrete a substance called **penicillinase.** The germs are then resistant in the ongoing battle against these penicillinase-producing bacteria. Protection can be provided, though, by adding a penicillin decoy. When the penicillinase attacks the decoy, it leaves the penicillin able to kill the bacteria. Examples of this penicillin and decoy strategy are amoxicillin + clavulanate *(Augmentin)* and ticarcillin + clavulanate *(Timentin).*

Although penicillins are usually very safe and well tolerated, there is the danger of penicillin allergy. Severe rashes can occur as a result of penicillin allergy. Other reactions can be life-threatening. A person can go into **anaphylaxis,** which is signaled by difficulty in breathing, swelling of the throat so as to cause suffocation, and shock symptoms. Persons who have penicillin allergies are asked to wear a medical ID to alert the medical staff in case emergency treatment is needed.

Cephalosporins. Cephalosporins are broad-spectrum, semisynthetic drugs related to penicillin. They can substitute for penicillin when germs have developed resistance. But people who are allergic to penicillin may be allergic to cephalosporins, too. Examples are cephalexin *(Keflex)* and cephalothin *(Keflin).*

Tetracyclines. The tetracyclines are broad-spectrum antibiotics. Examples of this drug group are tetracycline hydrochloride *(Achromycin V, Sumycin)* and doxycycline *(Vibramycin).*

Like the penicillins, the tetracyclines carry the danger of allergic reactions, superinfection, and the development of resistant organisms. They may also permanently discolor the developing teeth of children, cause stomach and liver problems, and cause a rash in patients exposed to sunlight (**photosensitivity**). Oral tetracyclines should not be given when a person is taking antacids or eating dairy products such as milk. Milk and antacids for stomach upset prevent the proper absorption of tetracyclines from the gastrointestinal tract.

Macrolides. Macrolides, such as erythromycin, work against many gram-positive cocci, as well as bacilli and rickettsiae. Because they kill many of the same germs as penicillin, macrolides are good substitutes to use for people with penicillin allergies. They are also used in the treatment of Legionnaires' disease. Although erythromycin is widely used, it does have drawbacks. It must be taken for up to four times a day, and it often causes stomach upset. Newer macrolides, including azithromycin *(Zithromax),* clarithromycin *(Biaxin),* and roxithromycin are less frequently dosed and are better tolerated then erythromycin.

Aminoglycosides. Aminoglycosides are a group of broad-spectrum antibiotics that keep germ cells from building proteins they need for growth. Examples are amikacin *(Amikin),* gentamicin *(Garamycin),* and tobramycin *(Tobrex, Nebcin),* which are given parenterally for systemic effects. They are also available as one ingredient in creams and ointments for topical use (e.g., *Neosporin, Cortisporin Otic)* and in oral forms for a local antibacterial effect (e.g., in preparing the intestines for bowel surgery). When given by injection, there is danger of nerve damage that can cause deafness. These drugs also can damage the kidneys. Aminoglycoside blood levels require close monitoring.

Sulfonamides. Sulfonamides, or sulfa drugs, are useful for many different types of infection. They can be given orally or topically. The combination of a sulfonamide, sulfamethoxazole, with trimethoprim makes a very powerful antibiotic regimen. It is so useful, in fact, that this combination has been given the name "cotrimoxazole," which is the active ingredient in the drugs *Bactrim* and *Septra*. Cotrimoxazole can be given orally or intravenously.

Side effects from sulfonamides are frequent. Common side effects are fever, rash, nausea, vomiting, and diarrhea. Low blood counts can also result from taking this medicine. Sulfonamides may cause crystals to form in the urine. This can cause urinary complications. For this reason, patients taking sulfa drugs should be given plenty of fluids each day.

Gamma Globulin

Gamma globulin is a protein that circulates in the bloodstream and contains the antibodies that make people immune to specific diseases. Because gamma globulin contains many different antibodies, it is sometimes given in large doses to patients in the hope of preventing an infection. For example, if a person has been exposed to viral hepatitis, a liver disease, the doctor might order several injections of gamma globulin to ward off the infection. Gamma globulin is also given to people whose bodies lack these substances from birth.

> ◆ **NOTES** ◆ ◆ ◆ ◆ ◆ ◆ ◆ ◆ ◆ ◆ ◆ ◆ ◆ ◆ ◆ ◆
>
> You should be familiar with drugs given in Table 6-3. Product information tables such as this appear in many of the remaining chapters of this text. You are not expected to memorize all of the information given. However, you should read them carefully. Your study of drugs in this text is designed to enable you to read and understand the latest drug information provided in drug references.

CANCER AND CHEMOTHERAPY

Cancer is not one disease but several hundred. The course of the disease and its treatment vary with the part of the body that is affected. In the remaining chapters, several forms of cancer are mentioned, along with the body systems or organs they affect. However, the drugs used to treat cancer are described here because they are best understood by looking at processes that take place at the cell level. They are also similar to antibiotics because they, too, destroy living cells.

All cancers have several features in common.

- *Rapid cell growth and reproduction.* This growth is caused by a change in the genetic code (or "messages") governing normal cell reproduction. These changes cause cancer cells to reproduce at a much faster rate than normal.

- *Effects on adjacent cells.* Cancer cells can invade nearby tissues as they grow, causing destruction.

- *Seeding.* Cancer cells can "seed" (implant) themselves in other parts of the body and start new growths there. This is called **metastasis.** We say that a cancer has metastasized to another part of the body.

Rapid cell growth may give rise to **tumors,** which are lumps or masses of tissue. Not all tumors are cancerous, however. Noncancerous tumors are called **benign** tumors. They involve rapid cell growth, but the cells do not invade nearby tissues or spread to other parts of the body.

TABLE 6-3: Anti-Infectives

Antibiotics
Penicillins
  Penicillin
  Ampicillin
  Amoxicillin
  Ampicillin/sulbactam (Unasyn)
  Amoxicillin/Clavulanate
    (Augmentin)
  Nafcillin
  Oxacillin
  Dicloxacillin
  Carbencillin (Geocillin)
  Ticarcillin (Ticar)
  Ticarcillin/clavulanate (Timentin)
  Azlocillin (Azlin)
  Mezlocillin (Mezlin)
  Piperacillin (Pipracil)
  Piperacillin/tazobactam
Fluoroquinolones
  Norfloxacin (Noroxin)
  Ciprofloxacin (Cipro)
  Ofloxacin (Floxin)
  Enoxacin (Penetrex)
  Temafloxacin (Omniflox)
  Clindamycin (Cleocin)
  Metronidazole (Flagyl)
  Vancomycin (Vancocin)
  Rifampin

Imipenem (Primaxin)
Aztreonam
Cephalosporins
  Cefazolin (Ancef, Kefzol)
  Cephalexin (Keflex)
  Cephradine (Velosef, Anspor)
  Cephalothin (Keflin)
  Cephadroxil (Duricef)
  Cefonicid (Monocid)
  Cefamandole (Mandol)
  Cefuroxime (Zinacef, Kefurox)
  Cefaclor (Celor)
  Cefuroxime axemil (Ceftin)
  Cefoxin (Mefoxin)
  Cefmetazole (Zefazone)
  Cefotetan (Cefotan)
  Cefotaxime (Claforan)
  Ceftizoxime (Cefizox)
  Ceftriaxone (Rocephin)
  Cefixime (Suprax)
  Cefoperazone (Cefobid)
  Cefrazidime (Fortaz, Tazicef)
Sulfonamides
  Sulfadiazine
  Sulfasoxazole (Gantrisin)
  Sulfamethoxazole/trimethoprim
    (Bactrim, Septra)

Aminoglycosides
  Gentamicin (Garamycin)
  Tobramycin (Tobrex, Nebcin)
  Amikacin (Amikin)
  Netilmicin (Netromycin)
  Streptomycin
  Kanamycin (Kantrex)
  Neomycin
Macrolides
  Erythromycin (ERYC), E-mycin,
    PCE, Ilosone EES
  Azithromycin (Zithromax)
  Clarithromycin (Biaxin)
  Roxithromycin
Tetracyclines
  Tetracycline hydrochloride
    (Achromycin V, Sumycin)
  Doxycycline (Vibramycin)
  Minocycline (Minocin)

Antivirals
  Acyclovir (Zovirax)
  Ganciclovir (Cytovene)
  Foscarnet (Foscarir)
  Zidovudine (Azt) (Retrovir)
  Didanosine (ddl) (Videx)
  Dideoxyctidine (ddC) (Hivid)
  Ribavirin (Virazole)
  Amantadine (Symmetrel)

Cancerous tumors are called **malignant** tumors. As they grow, they put pressure on surrounding healthy tissues and organs and also invade them, causing destruction. Some cancers affect whole systems, such as the blood and lymph-forming organs, rather than causing a local tumor. In such cases the cancer cells circulate throughout the body.

Early detection of cancer gives the best chance of curing the disease. The methods of treatment most often used first are surgery and radiation. Surgery is employed to remove tumors and nearby lymph glands, where cancer cells that have spread from the tumor may be trapped. Radiation may be focused on a specific spot to kill the cancer cells. It may also be implanted in nearby tissue or swallowed in a substance that is attracted to the site of the cancer.

Drugs for Chemotherapy

Drug treatment of cancer is called **chemotherapy.** Drugs can cure a few rare types of cancer, but they are more often used to control cancer symptoms after surgery and radiation have failed to bring about a cure. They also are used in system-wide invasions of cancer cells, such as leukemia and Hodgkin's disease.

The drugs used for chemotherapy are powerful and have strong effects on healthy cells as well as cancer cells. They are dangerous drugs whose use has to be carefully planned and supervised by a physician. Some of them are specifically attracted to cells that are multiplying rapidly. Thus they rush to the scene of a tumorous growth, killing cancer cells.

But at the same time, they are attracted to the blood-forming centers of the body because there the cells are also multiplying rapidly. When the drugs kill blood cells, they weaken the body and destroy some of its defenses. Patients receiving chemotherapy often bruise easily because many platelets (parts of the blood that help stop bleeding) have been destroyed. They may be especially prone to infection because of the destruction of white blood cells. Their bones may heal slowly and also may break easily because the cancer drugs weaken the bone tissue where blood cells are produced.

Other areas of the body that have rapidly multiplying cells are the skin and the linings of the mouth, throat, stomach, and intestines. These areas, too, are affected by chemotherapy. Side effects such as nausea, vomiting, and hair loss are common.

Doses must be carefully controlled because large doses can be toxic to healthy cells. Often some toxic effects are necessary to achieve the benefit of a drug's cancer-suppressing ability. Rather than giving a low dose continuously over a long period of time, cancer drugs are sometimes given in cycles—intensive treatment followed by a recovery period of 4–6 weeks, followed by another intensive treatment, and so on. This gives the body time to recover from the toxic effects and to build blood cells back up to a normal level.

No drug is able to kill all cancer cells at one time. But each successive dose kills a few more, so that the population is kept down to a level where the symptoms are under control. The effect of chemotherapy is shown in Figure 6-5, which depicts the reproductive life of a cancer cell. Without chemotherapy, after six generations this cell would have produced 64 cancer

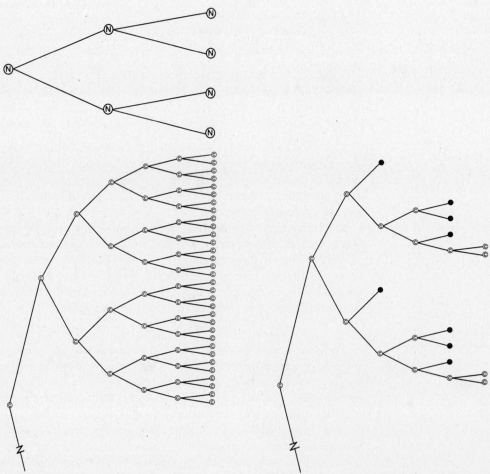

Figure 6-5 Compare the reproduction of cancer cells and normal cells. Chemotherapy slows reproduction by destroying some of the abnormal cells.

cells. With two waves of chemotherapy, it produced only six. During the same amount of time, a normal cell might have reproduced itself only one or two times.

Remission means the disappearance of symptoms (not just of cancer, but of any disease). The object of cancer chemotherapy is to bring about remission and to keep the symptoms from recurring. Chemotherapy is not guaranteed to cure cancer, but it can give the patient many more years of useful life.

Drugs used against cancer are called **antineoplastics** (Figure 6-6). The prefix *anti-* means against, and *neoplasm* means tumor. These drugs slow down or kill growing cells by interfering with chemical processes or by substituting for nutrients in the cells so the cells "starve" to death. Other terms used for anticancer drugs are cytostatic, which means that they stop all growth, and cytotoxic, which means poisonous to cells.

Alkylating Agents (Nitrogen Mustards). Alkylating agents are drugs that chemically latch onto important cell parts so that they do not work properly. This results in cell destruction. Nitrogen mustards are related to mustard gas, first used in World War I as a chemical weapon. Applied to the skin, as in a "mustard bomb," they blister the skin. But used as cancer drugs, they stop the growth of many cancer cells. Alkylating agents have toxic effects on the blood-building organs, the gastrointestinal system, and the sex glands. An immediate side effect is usually vomiting and nausea. But after a while, the patient's daily blood counts will reveal that fewer lymph cells are being produced in the bone marrow, signaling remission. Examples of alkylating agents are mechlorethamine hydrochloride *(Mustargen)*, chlorambucil *(Leukeran)*, and cyclophosphamide *(Cytoxan)*.

A newer type of alkylating agent is a group of drugs called nitrosoureas (carmustine and lomustine). These drugs are able to pass into the brain, making them useful for treating brain tumors.

Antimetabolites. Antimetabolites interfere with metabolism. Metabolism is the cell process that burns nutrients to produce energy for growth and action. Antimetabolites look very much like the normal nutrients that cells use, but they cannot produce energy. The cancer cells consume them, but since the antimetabolites do not provide energy, the cell eventually dies. This is similar to the action of sulfonamides on bacteria and viruses. Examples of antimetabolites are fluorouracil, mercaptopurine, and cytarabine *(Cyto-sar-U)*.

Antibiotics. Some antibiotics stop the growth of cancer cells and so are used in chemotherapy. Examples are dactinomycin *(Cosmegen)*, bleomycin, doxorubicin *(Adriamycin)*, and plicamycin *(Mithracin)*.

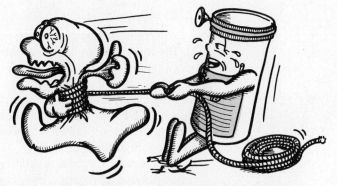

Figure 6-6 Antineoplastics destroy or slow the growth of cancer cells.

Hormones. Sex hormones (e.g., estrogen, testosterone) are used to control specific cancers in the sex organs, such as cancer of the breast, prostate, and uterus. Examples of these are dromostanolone *(Drolban)* and fluoxymesterone *(Halotestin)*. Other hormones suppress the production of lymph cells and make the patient feel better, so they are used in managing leukemia.

Note that the described antineoplastics may be given in various combinations. The drugs vincristine *(Oncovin)* and vinblastine *(Velban)* are sometimes included in these combinations. They are products of the periwinkle plant (vinca), and they work by interfering with cell division. See the product information chart at the end of this unit for representative antineoplastics and their uses, actions, doses, and side effects.

One of the most exciting new areas of drug therapy is called **biotechnology**, or biogenetic engineering. Microscopic substances, such as proteins, that are normally made in the human body are found and captured. Biotechnology now allows these substances to be made in large quantities in the laboratory. They can then be used to help control the immune system of patients, as well as those with infections or transplanted organs.

The name of some of these products include tumor necrosis factor (TNF), anti-TNF, monoclonal antibodies, interleukin-1 (IL-1), and colony-stimulating factor (CSF). For example, CSFs are proteins normally produced by the body that trigger the production of more blood cells. G-CFS *(Neupogen)* or GM-CSF *(Leukine* or *Prokine)* can be given to cancer patients with low blood counts caused by chemotherapy. These drugs, which are given by injection only, are very expensive.

Care of the Cancer Patient

Patients undergoing chemotherapy need special care and emotional support from you. They must deal not only with the threat of cancer itself, but also with the unpleasant, often dangerous side effects of chemotherapy. Many of the drugs given for cancer therapy must be administered parenterally by specially trained nurses or by physicians. However, you may be involved in giving some of the routine drugs for pain and nausea. You can provide emotional support by listening to your patients' fears and needs and by doing what you can to help make them comfortable. You should also observe them carefully for physical signs of drug side effects and disease effects, especially:

- nausea and vomiting
- irritation of the mucous membranes of the mouth and throat
- signs of developing infections, especially around the eyes, nose, and rectum
- pain caused by the disease that could be treated with analgesics (pain relievers)
- fluid retention
- diarrhea
- fever

Chart these observations and follow the physician's orders.

Because antineoplastics irritate the gastrointestinal tract, from the mouth through the rectum, patients have trouble eating because it is uncomfortable. They may develop a painful inflammation of the mucous membranes of the mouth, called stomatitis. Encourage them to eat by providing a pleasant atmosphere and letting them select their own foods. Help with their oral hygiene by rinsing their mouths often with water or mouthwashes. Clean the teeth and gums gently with a soft brush.

Finally, take special care not to infect chemotherapy patients with germs from other patients. Remember, their bodies' natural defenses against infection may be seriously weakened by the antineoplastics they are taking.

ISOLATION PROCEDURES

There are two basic situations in which isolation procedures may be used:

- when a patient must be protected from any germs that you carry
- when you must be protected from any germs the patient is carrying (Figure 6-7).

Depending on the specific disease or germ danger, there are special types of isolation requiring different precautions.

Strict Isolation

The patient is kept in a separate room, with the door closed. All involved staff wear protective gowns, masks, and gloves. Hands must be washed upon entering and leaving the room. All equipment for drug administration must be discarded in special containers after use or must be disinfected and sterilized.

This type of isolation is ordered for hospital staph infections and serious infectious diseases that can be spread by touch and by air. It protects the medical staff (and other patients) from germs the patient is carrying.

Respiratory Isolation

The patient is kept in a separate room, with the door closed. Staff members wear protective masks only. Hands must be washed upon entering and leaving the room. Gloves are not necessary, but any object that is contaminated with fluids from the patient's nose and lungs must be disinfected so that the patient's germs are not spread to others. Meningitis, mumps, and tuberculosis are diseases requiring respiratory isolation.

Reverse Isolation (Protective Isolation)

The patient is kept in a separate room, with the door closed. Gown, mask, and gloves must be worn by the staff. Hands must be washed upon entering and leaving the room.

This type of isolation protects patients who have no immunity or who have weakened immunity because of leukemia or cancer chemotherapy; the patient is being protected from germs you are carrying.

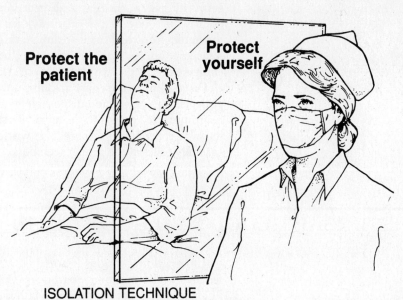

Protect the patient

Protect yourself

ISOLATION TECHNIQUE

Figure 6-7 Isolation technique—hand washing, gown, gloves, mask, cap, and disinfection of equipment—forms a barrier to germs.

Special procedures are also followed when handling patients with disease germs that pass out of the body in the feces (enteric precautions); burns and skin infections (wound and skin precautions); and open sores, blood infections, and draining wounds (discharge precautions). These do not require a separate room for the patient, but aseptic procedures must be followed to avoid causing or spreading infection.

Before administering drugs to any isolation patient, you should review isolation procedures in your agency's procedure manual or in a good nursing manual. The steps are specific and should be followed. There are usually instructions for putting on and taking off gowns, masks, and gloves and for disposing of materials and equipment.

The procedure you will most often be using, whether working with an isolation patient or not, is washing your hands. This is done both before and after administering a medication. Practice Procedure 6-1 at the end of this chapter will help refresh your memory of the proper hand-washing technique.

When administering medications to an isolation patient, you may wonder which items are considered contaminated. The answer is everything that has been in direct or indirect contact with the patient. An example of indirect contact would be your touching a glass that has remained near a coughing patient, even if the patient had never actually touched the glass. Your gown and mask protect you (or the patient) from indirect contact. Your gloves protect you from direct contact. For additional protection, you may ask patients to take their own medications and dispose of supplies while you watch, as long as they are able to do this.

When working with a patient who has an infectious disease, it may be helpful to know the main places where germs can be picked up. Germs leave the body of a diseased person in the secretions of the nose and mouth; in material coughed up from the lungs; in the feces or anything touched by feces (bedclothes, toilet, etc.); in the urine; in the vaginal area; in drainage from infected wounds; and in the blood (in the case of hepatitis). Those sources of contamination are the ones toward which aseptic and isolation procedures are directed.

You may take advantage of disposable materials to avoid carrying germs from one place to another. Where disposable materials are not available or not practical (as with permanent pieces of equipment), contaminated items must be washed and sterilized by using a special machine. Machines can kill germs by baking them at high heat, searing them with steam, or bombarding them with sound waves or ultraviolet rays. A common sterilizing machine is the **autoclave,** which uses steam. A variety of chemical germ killers called **disinfectants** are also available for sterilizing surgical tools and other pieces of equipment.

Disposal procedures are also important when you are working with infected patients. Equipment and disposable materials must be specially wrapped before being discarded or sent to the hospital's sterilization unit. Each agency usually has its own proper disposal procedures written up in a procedure manual. Study these carefully to learn the proper techniques.

◆◆
UNIVERSAL BLOOD AND BODY FLUID PRECAUTIONS

Universal precautions means that all patients are considered potentially infectious with blood-borne pathogens. Examples are hepatitis B virus (HBV) and human immunodeficiency virus (HIV), the virus that causes AIDS. Health care workers are exposed to these pathogens primarily through mucous membranes, nonintact skin, and needlesticks.

Blood is the most important vehicle for transmission of these pathogens. Other body fluids that can be involved are cerebrospinal (CSF), synovial (joint), pleural (lung), peritoneal (abdominal), and amniotic fluids; semen; vaginal secretions; and human breast milk. Gloves and other protective clothing should be used routinely in handling contaminated needles and other sharp instruments. Table 6-4 lists the universal blood and body fluid precautions. These guidelines are frequently revised, so be sure your facility has the current, up-to-date guidelines in use.

TABLE 6-4: Universal Blood and Body Fluid Precautions

Employer: Protect Health Care Worker
- Explain activities that expose workers to blood-borne pathogens.
- Develop standard operating procedures to prevent worker exposure.
- Provide initial and ongoing education on universal precautions.
- Follow up worker compliance with guidelines.
- Redesign the workplace and modify the workplace environment.

Health Care Worker: Use Appropriate Barrier Precautions
- Wear gloves to reduce blood contamination to skin surface.
- Wash hands/skin immediately when exposed.
- Change and discard punctured or torn gloves.
- Wear mask, gowns, and eye/face shields to protect mucous membranes.
- Do not work if you have dermatitis or exudative lesions.
- If pregnant, do not risk exposing the fetus to blood-borne pathogens by lack of precautions.

Health Care Worker: Prevent Needlestick Injuries
- Do not break, bend, or remove needles by hand from syringes.
- Do not recap needles if avoidable.
- Place disposable needles in puncture-resistant containers.
- Place these containers as close to the work area as possible.
- Place nondisposable needles and equipment in puncture-resistant containers and transport them to the processing area.
- Transport contaminated equipment to the appropriate area.

CATEGORY, NAME[a] AND ROUTE	USES AND DISEASES	ACTIONS	USUAL DOSE[b] AND ADMINISTRATION	SIDE EFFECTS AND ADVERSE REACTIONS
Antibiotics				
Penicillin G *(various)* IV, IM, po	Pneumonia, syphilis, strep throat, etc.	Inhibits bacterial cell wall synthesis	5–20 million units/day; watch patient closely for allergic reaction	Hypersensitivity reactions such as rash, chills, shortness of breath
Vancomycin *(Vancocin)* IV, po	Staph infections, antibiotic-associated diarrhea	Inhibits bacterial cell wall synthesis	1 g IV q12h infused slowly over at least 1 hour (not for IM use)	Red man syndrome, muscle spasms, low blood pressure, painful if given IM, hearing loss
Gentamicin *(Garamycin)* IV, IM	Bloodstream infections, urinary tract infections	Blocks protein synthesis	80 mg IV q8hr; based on patient's weight and kidney function	Kidney damage, hearing loss, upset of balance; drug levels must be closely monitored
Cotrimoxazole *(Septra, Bactrim)* IV, po	Pneumonia, bronchitis, urinary tract infections	Blocks folate metabolism pathway	One double-strength tablet po q12h; encourage fluids	Nausea, vomiting, diarrhea, rash, allergic reaction to sulfa, liver damage
Ciprofloxacin *(Cipro)* po	Pneumonia, bone infection, urinary tract infection	Inhibits DNA gyrase	500 mg po q12hr; do not take with antacids	Headache, stomach upset, oral thrush
Antifungals				
Amphotericin B *(Fungizone)* IV	Systemic fungal infections	Damages fungal cell wall	20–50 mg IV daily (after 1-mg test dose); Infuse over 4–6 hours	Fever, chills, nausea, kidney damage, vein irritation
Antivirals				
Acyclovir *(Zovirax)* IV, po, top	Herpes simplex, chickenpox, shingles	Stops viral replication	250–500 mg IV q8hr; 200–800 mg po 5x/day	Kidney damage, headache, confusion, irritability, stomach upset

a   Product names given in parentheses are examples only. Check current drug references for a complete listing of available products.

b   Average adult doses given. However, dosages are determined by a physician and vary with the purpose of the therapy and the particular patient. The doses presented here are for general information only.

◆◆

Representative Antineoplastics ◆ ◆ ◆ ◆

CATEGORY, NAME[a] AND ROUTE	USES AND DISEASES	ACTIONS	USUAL DOSE[b] AND SPECIAL INSTRUCTIONS	SIDE EFFECTS AND ADVERSE REACTIONS
Alkylating Agents				
Mechlorethamine (Mustargen)	Hodgkin's disease, lymphosarcoma	Inhibits rapidly growing cells	IV dosage according to body weight, adjusted to highest nontoxic dose; assist patient with oral hygiene; give adequate fluid; follow physician's orders carefully; note length of time for IV infusion; watch for pain at infusion site	Nausea, vomiting, bleeding, bruising
Carmustine (BiNCU)	Brain tumor, Hodgkin's disease, lymphomas	Inhibits of cell synthesis	IV dosage according to surface area, pain at injection site common	Blood and liver problems, nausea, vomiting
Antimetabolites				
Fluorouracil (Adrucil)	Cancer of the breast colon, rectum, stomach, and pancreas	Slows reproduction of cells	IV dosage according to body weight; avoid extravasation	Loss of appetite, nausea, vomiting, stomatitis, diarrhea, fever, bleeding, sore throat
Mercaptopurine (Purinethol)	Leukemias	Slows reproduction of cells	Oral dosage according to body weight, adjusted to highest nontoxic dose	Blood and liver problems
Antibiotics				
Dactinomycin (Cosmegen)	Cancer of the testes and uterus, Wilms' tumor	Inhibits cell reproduction	IV dosage according to body weight, adjusted to highest nontoxic dose. Drug is corrosive; avoid contact with skin; avoid extravasation	Nausea, vomiting, fever, stomatitis, bleeding, bruising, loss of hair
Hormones				
Dromostanolone (Drolban)	Cancer of the breast	Tumor regression, promotes feeling of well-being in advanced cancer	100 mg IM three times per week	Mild virilism (deepening) voice, growth of facial hair), hypercalcemia

[a] Product names given in parentheses are examples only. Check current drug references for a complete listing of available products.

[b] Average adult doses are given. However, dosages are determined by a physician and vary with the purpose of the therapy and the particular patient. The doses presented here are for general information only.

• • • PRACTICE PROCEDURE 6-1 • • •

Administering Medication to an Isolation Patient

> ◆ **NOTE** ◆ ◆ ◆ ◆ ◆ ◆ ◆ ◆ ◆ ◆ ◆ ◆ ◆ ◆ ◆ ◆ ◆
>
> You may wish to practice the procedure several times using a different type of isolation each time.

Equipment

- Medication order for an oral medication to be taken with water
- Kardex, medication record, patient chart
- Oral medication (e.g., tetracycline capsule)
- Medication tray or cart with souffle cups
- Gown, mask, and gloves
- Instructions for basic isolation procedures in your agency's procedure manual
- Water pitcher and glass (next to patient's bed)

Procedure

1. Assemble equipment. Use disposable equipment if possible.
2. Read medication order and set up medication. Check to see that you have the RIGHT DOSE of the RIGHT MEDICATION for the RIGHT PATIENT by the RIGHT ROUTE at the RIGHT TIME.
3. Check to see what kind of isolation the patient is under—respiratory, strict, reverse, or special precautions (enteric, skin wounds, discharge, etc.). There should be a sign on the door of the patient's room or on the Kardex telling the type of isolation.
4. Review isolation procedures for the specific type of isolation and decide what clothing you must wear—gown, mask, and/or gloves. Here is a brief reminder:
   - *For reverse isolation.* Wear gown, mask, and gloves. This provides protection for the patient.
   - *For respiratory isolation.* Wear a mask only. This protects you from airborne bacteria that may be inhaled into the lungs.
   - *For strict isolation.* Wear gown, mask, and gloves. This provides protection for you, since you must not touch anything contaminated.
     But remember to wash your hands before you put on the protective clothing.
5. Wash your hands, following standard nursing practice. In other words, use soap and water to make a lather and then scrub each finger and the front and back of each hand with a circular motion. Rinse, keeping hands lower than elbows so that water flows from the cleaner area toward the dirtier area. Lather and rinse again. The washing process should last for at least 1–2 minutes. Dry hands with a paper towel, using the same elbow-to-hand motion.
6. Now put on your gown, mask, and/or gloves, following the proper procedure.
7. Carry the medication into the patient's room in a souffle cup or envelope. Leave the drug cart or tray outside the door.
8. Identify the patient, following agency procedure. Explain what you are going to do (e.g., give the patient an antibiotic to help heal an infection or fight disease germs). If necessary, assist the patient into a comfortable position for taking the medication.

9. Administer the medication. Have the patient pour a glass of water from the bedside pitcher and then take the medication from the souffle cup and swallow it with water while you watch.

10. Give any special instructions regarding the medication, for example, mild side effects that may be expected. Make the patient comfortable before leaving the room.

11. Remove gown, mask, and/or gloves and discard according to the rules of your agency. Wash your hands, following standard nursing practice. Use a paper towel to turn off the water faucet, unless there is a foot or knee pedal.

12. Chart the medication, noting the time, dose, and anything unusual that you may have noticed or that the patient may have mentioned.

Demonstrate this procedure for your instructor or the nurse in charge.

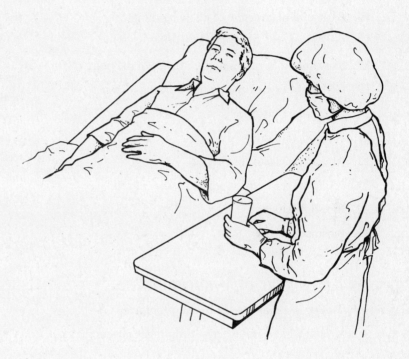

CHAPTER 6 REVIEW

Using Medical Terminology

Define each of the terms listed below.

1. Antibody _____

2. Immunization _____

3. Pathogen _____

4. Leukocyte _____

5. Chemotherapy _____

6. Biostatic _____

7. Biocidal _____

8. Malignant _____

9. Hypersensitivity _____

10. Biotechnology _____

11. HBV _____

12. HIV _____

13. AIDS _____

14. Penicillinase _____

15. Biotechnology _____

Match the characteristic or description to the appropriate term.

_____ 16. Basic unit of structure of all living things

_____ 17. Groups of cells working together

_____ 18. Substance that makes up two-thirds of the body

_____ 19. Groups of organs and tissues working together

_____ 20. Fluid found inside cells

_____ 21. Fluid surrounding cells

_____ 22. Ability of cells to split in two

_____ 23. Ability of the body to replace damaged cells

_____ 24. Biocidal activity

_____ 25. Biostatic activity

a. tissues
b. water
c. cells
d. systems
e. healing
f. reproduction
g. cytoplasm
h. tissue fluid
i. inhibit growth
j. kill

Acquiring Knowledge of Medications

Answer the following questions in the spaces provided.

26. List two ways in which anti-infective drugs fight infection. _____

_____

_____

27. Which parts of the body may be damaged by aminoglycosides? _____

_____

_____

28. What is another name for erythromycin? _____

_____

29. Name three characteristics of cancer cells. _____

_____

_____

_____

30. Antineoplastics harm healthy cells as well as cancer cells. Which parts of the body are especially affected by chemotherapy?

_____

_____

_____

31. Why might a physician order a Gram stain? _____

_____

32. Why are isolation procedures used? _____

_____

33. List the three main types of isolation (in which patients are kept in separate rooms). _____

_____

_____

_____

Match these anti-infectives to their descriptions.

_____ **34.** Semisynthetic forms of penicillin

_____ **35.** Broad-spectrum antibiotics that should not be taken with antacids or milk

_____ **36.** Semisynthetic drugs that can substitute for penicillin when germs have developed resistance

_____ **37.** Broad-spectrum antibiotics that can cause nerve damage

_____ **38.** Synthetic drugs used mostly for urinary tract infections

_____ **39.** Blood protein containing antibodies, given to protect the body from infection

_____ **40.** Substitute for penicillin, used in Legionnaires' disease

a. tetracyclines

b. cephalosporins

c. sulfonamides

d. ampicillin, amoxicillin

e. kanamycin, gentamicin

f. macrolides

g. gamma globulin

Match these terms to their descriptions.

_____ **41.** Laboratory test to identify germs

_____ **42.** Laboratory test to determine which drug will kill a specific germ

_____ **43.** Drugs that affect many pathogens

_____ **44.** Drugs that affect only a few pathogens

_____ **45.** A germ's immunity to the effects of germ-killing drugs

_____ **46.** Allergiclike reaction to a drug after taking several doses

a. narrow spectrum

b. resistance

c. Gram stain

d. broad spectrum

e. hypersensitivity

f. culture and sensitivity test

Applying Knowledge on the Job

Answer the following questions in the spaces provided.

47. Why are staph and other infections a special problem in hospitals and long-term care units? Give at least three reasons.

_____

_____

_____

_____

_____

48. List three ways in which a health care worker can be exposed to HBV and HIV. _____

_____

_____

_____

49. List at least three possible problems associated with the use of penicillin. _____

_____

_____

_____

50. You have just administered penicillin to Mrs. Mosley. Within minutes she goes into shock, has difficulty breathing, and shows signs of swelling in the throat. What is probably the matter, and what should you do?

_____

_____

_____

51. Why should oral tetracyclines not be given to a patient taking antacids or dairy products? _____

_____

_____

_____

52. What signs should you look for when giving medications to cancer patients? _____

_____

_____

_____

53. When should you wash your hands during medication administration? _____

_____

54. List at least three ways in which germs leave the body of an infected person. _____

_____

_____

_____

55. Where should you look to find the proper procedures for isolation and disposal of contaminated materials?

_____

_____

_____

Match these types of antineoplastics to examples and descriptions.

_____ **56.** Alkylating agents

_____ **57.** Antimetabolites

_____ **58.** Antibiotics used against cancer

_____ **59.** Sex hormones

a. used especially to fight cancer of the prostate, uterus, and breast

b. take the place of nutrients in cancer cells

c. bleomycin and dactinomycin

d. nitrogen mustard and mechlorethamine

Using Resources on the Job

Obtain a current copy of the PDR from your school, nursing unit, or clinic. Use it to answer the following questions in a notebook or on index cards.

60. Use the PDR, Section 4, Generic and Chemical Name Index, to find another product name for each drug listed on the Representative Drug List on pages 144–145 of this chapter.

61. In Section 3, Product Category Index of the PDR, find the subheading antimetabolites. List all the drugs named.

62. Section 3, Product Category Index, of the PDR gives a page number for some drugs shown in Section 5, Product Identification Section. Using these page numbers, identify the pictures of those drugs shown as antimetabolites.

63. Notice the different forms Section 5 displays for two products. If solid, state the form. If liquid, how is it administered?

64. For the same two drugs you identified in the previous question, name the manufacturer. In Section 1 of the PDR, Manufacturer's Index, find the address of the manufacturer.

65. In Section 2 of the PDR, Product Name Index, identify the pages that give detailed information about these two drugs. Read about these two drugs in Section 6, Product Information.

66. In Section 6 of the PDR, under *Dosage and Administration,* write out the information referring to children and the elderly.

67. In Section 7 of the PDR, Diagnostic Product Information, find the name of the manufacturer that produced the two drugs you identified in Question 63.

68. List the diagnostic drugs produced by one of the manufacturers you identified in the previous question.

69. Write a summary of this exercise below.

_____
_____
_____
_____
_____
_____
_____
_____
_____
_____
_____
_____
_____

If you have a problem answering any of the above questions, look in the back of the PDR under *Discontinued Products* to see if any of the drugs are listed there.

Using Medical Terminology

1. Substance produced in the body to kill specific germs

2. Shot or vaccination to stimulate antibody formation against a certain disease germ

3. Harmful germ, one that can cause infection

4. White blood cell specialized to swallow germs

5. Drug therapy for cancer symptoms

6. Ability to inhibit growth of microorganisms

7. Ability to kill microorganisms

8. Cancerous

9. Symptoms relating to anaphylaxis

10. The ability to make proteins that are normally found in the body

11. Hepatitis B virus

12. HIV, the virus that causes AIDS

13. Acquired Immune Deficiency Syndrome

14. Enzyme produced by microbes that makes them resistant to penicillin

15. Biogenic engineering, the ability to make proteins that are normally produced in the body

16. c   17. a   18. b   19. d

20. g   21. h   22. f   23. e

24. j   25. i

Acquiring Knowledge of Medications

26. By killing terms directly and by slowing the growth of germs.

27. There is a risk of nerve damage that can cause deafness; the kidneys.

28. Macrolides.

29. They grow and divide more rapidly than normal cells. They invade nearby healthy tissues. They metastasize (spread) to other parts of the body.

30. Parts of the body where cells are dividing rapidly, such as the blood-forming areas of the bones.

31. The results of a Gram stain determine the choice of an antibiotic that will be most effective for a specific pathogen.

32. Isolation procedures protect the patient from germs that health care workers are carrying and protect health care workers from germs that the patient is carrying.

33. Strict, respiratory, and reverse (protective).

34. d   35. a   36. b   37. e   38. c

39. g   40. f   41. c   42. f   43. d

44. a   45. b   46. e

Applying Knowledge on the Job

47. Infections in hospitals are dangerous because drug-resistant germs that live in some health facilities cannot be killed by antibiotics. In hospitals, a large number of at-risk patients are gathered into one place. Patients with skin wounds and lowered resistance are easily attacked by germs. Medical staff can carry germs from patient to patient as they work.

48. a. Through mucous membranes
    b. Through nonintact skin
    c. By needlesticks

49. Allergic reaction; superinfection; some penicillins are poorly absorbed by the oral route and/or excreted quickly; microbes develop resistance by secreting penicillinase.

50. The patient is probably allergic to penicillin and is going into anaphylactic shock. You should get emergency help immediately.

51. Antacids and dairy products prevent the proper absorption of tetracyclines from the gastrointestinal tract.

52. Gastrointestinal upset (nausea, vomiting, diarrhea), pain, fever, and infections.

53. Before and after leaving the room or before and after giving medication.

54. Secretions from the nose and mouth; secretions coughed up from lungs; feces or anything touched by feces; drainage from wounds; infected blood.

55. In your agency's procedure manual; if they do not have one, look in a good nursing manual.

56. d   57. b   58. c   59. a

Using Resources on the Job

60–68. Answers will vary depending on the edition of the PDR that is used.

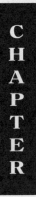
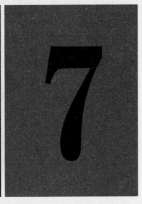

Drugs for the Skin

◆◆ In this chapter you will learn about the structure of the skin and its functions. You will study major skin disorders, the medical terms for their symptoms, and the drugs used to treat them. You will learn to administer topical drugs to the skin with a proper understanding of their uses and action.

COMPETENCIES

After studying this chapter, you should be able to

- name the three layers of skin tissue and the structures contained in each.
- list the main functions of the integumentary system.
- name the secretions of the ceruminous, sebaceous, sudoriferous, and mammary glands.
- state the normal body temperature.
- explain the process of inflammation.
- list and define the common symptoms of skin disorders.
- describe the major skin disorders.
- state the actions and give examples of the following topical medication categories: keratolytics, protectives, astringents, antipruritics, topical corticosteroids, vasoconstrictor/venous insufficiency treatments, anti-infectives, antiseptics, topical anesthetics, and parasiticides.
- list five ways of increasing absorption of drugs into the skin layers.
- follow general instructions for administering topical medications to the skin (psychological support, preparing the patient, bandaging, etc.).
- follow the correct procedures for applying topical creams, lotions, liniments, ointments, and aerosol sprays.

VOCABULARY

acne: skin condition caused by pores plugged with sebum

antifungal: drug that kills or prevents the growth of fungi; also called fungicide

antihistamine: drug that lessens the effects of histamine

anti-inflammatory: drug that suppresses inflammation

antipruritic: drug that relieves itching

antiseptic: drug that destroys germs on skin surfaces

ceruminous glands: sweat glands in the ear that secrete ear wax

contact dermatitis: reaction to an irritating substance that has touched the skin

corticosteroids: drugs used on the skin because they suppress inflammation, tighten the blood vessels, and relieve itching

dandruff: noninflammatory irritation of the scalp

decubitus ulcers: bedsores

dermatitis: inflammation of the skin causing bumps, blisters, scales, or scabs; also called eczema

dermis: middle layer of skin

disinfectant: agent used to kill germs on surgical instruments

ecchymosis: escape of blood into tissues from ruptured blood vessels; causes a bruise

eczema: also called dermatitis

edema: swelling

epidermis: outer skin layer

erythema: reddening of the skin

fungus: one-celled, plantlike parasite (plural: fungi)

hair follicle: a structure of the skin from which hair grows

histamine: substance normally present in the body; actively released in response to tissue injury

hives: welts

inflammation: the body's reaction to irritation; a process that results in swelling, reddening, heat, and pain

integument: the skin

keratin: protein contained in cells of the epidermis, nails, hair, and horny tissue

keratolytic: drug that destroys keratin and promotes peeling

keratosis: buildup and hardening of keratin in the skin

lesion: sore, break, or any abnormal place on the skin (in general, any detrimental changes in the structure of a body part)

macerate: soften by moistening, causing increased absorption through the skin

mammary glands: sweat glands that secrete milk, located in the female breasts

occlusive bandage: bandage that seals in drugs, body heat, and moisture

parasite: organism that lives on or in another organism (e.g., lice, mites, tapeworms)

parasiticide: drug that kills parasites

pediculicide: drug that kills lice

pediculosis: infection caused by lice

petechiae: tiny, purplish-red spots on the skin due to bleeding in the skin layers

photodermatitis: irritation caused by skin sensitivity to light

protective: drug that soothes, cools, and protects inflamed skin

pruritus: itching

psoriasis: chronic skin disease of unknown cause; involves drying and scaling of skin

scabicide: drug that kills mites

scabies: infection caused by mites

scaling: an excess of keratin in the epidermis

sebaceous glands: glands in the skin that produce oil

seborrheic dermatitis: inflammatory irritation of the scalp, face, or groin producing greasy scales

sebum: oil that lubricates the skin, produced by the sebaceous glands

sense receptor: structure that picks up sensations of hot, cold, touch, pain, or pressure in the skin

subcutaneous: deepest skin layer, made up of fatty tissue

sudoriferous glands: glands that produce sweat

transdermal delivery system: system in which drugs in patch form are absorbed into the bloodstream through the skin

transdermal/transcutaneous: passing, entering, or penetrating the skin

ulceration: open sore

vasoconstrictive drugs: drugs that tighten blood vessels in the area of the inflammation and reduce swelling

INTEGUMENTARY SYSTEM

The integumentary system consists of the skin (the **integument**), along with the hairs, nails, and glands that are embedded in it. The skin has been called the largest organ of the body because its surface area is so large. It forms a waterproof, protective covering for the entire body, but protection is not its only function.

The skin also senses changes in the environment, and it helps to regulate body temperature. The body's normal temperature is about 98.6°F (37°C). This is the temperature at which the cells maintain their normal functioning. Changes of even a few degrees above or below this normal temperature can disrupt body processes.

The skin actually consists of three distinct layers: the epidermis, the dermis, and the subcutaneous layer (Figure 7-1).

Epidermis

The outermost layer, the **epidermis**, is made of flat, tough epithelial cells that are constantly being shed and replaced. These cells contain the pigments that give

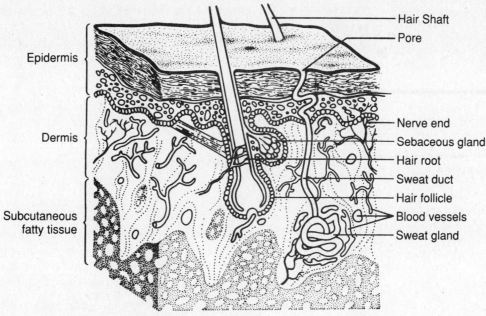

Figure 7-1 Cross section showing the three layers of the skin.

a person's skin its characteristic color. The epidermis forms a barrier against bacteria and moisture. It also holds water in to keep body tissues from drying out.

Any break in the epidermis, such as a puncture or a cut, lets in bacteria that may attack the deeper tissues. For this reason, all skin wounds must be kept clean until they heal.

Dermis

Just beneath the epidermis lies a second layer, the **dermis.** The dermis is made up of connective tissue interwoven with tiny blood vessels and nerve endings. It also contains several other structures:

- **Hair follicles,** from which grow the tiny hairs that cover the body.
- **Sebaceous glands,** or oil glands, that lubricate the hairs with oil or **sebum.**
- **Sudoriferous glands,** or sweat glands, that help regulate body temperature.
- **Sense receptors,** which send messages to the brain when they feel pain, pressure, heat, cold, touch, and so on.

Two glands in the dermal layer have very specific locations: **ceruminous glands** in the ear secrete ear wax, and **mammary glands** in the female breast secrete milk. These are both specialized forms of sweat glands.

Subcutaneous Layer

The **subcutaneous** layer is a combination of fibrous and fatty connective tissue. The fibrous tissue attaches the upper skin layers to the skeletal muscles. The fatty tissue holds in body heat and acts as an insulator against cold. It also acts as a storage area for energy in the form of fat. Some of the glands, follicles, and sense receptors in the dermis extend down into this subcutaneous layer.

SKIN DISORDERS

The skin reflects the upheavals inside the body caused by infectious diseases, such as measles and chickenpox, and by irritating substances that have been touched, swallowed, or inhaled. The skin is also a mirror of human emotions, which reveal themselves through blushing, paleness, and rashes.

This section describes disorders that are confined mainly to the skin area itself. However, the symptoms are similar, whether caused by systemic diseases or by local irritation. The symptoms are the result of the body's natural response to injury: **inflammation.**

Inflammation is a process that occurs wherever and whenever there is cell damage. The capillaries around the damaged area expand to bring in the white blood cells (the leukocytes), which are the germ fighters, and cell repair is begun. The "battle zone" is characterized by redness, swelling, heat, and pain. The person experiencing this reaction, may be very uncomfortable, but the inflammatory process is essential for survival.

Major Skin Diseases

The diseases and conditions that cause these symptoms are numerous. A few of the most common conditions will be described.

Contact Dermatitis. Contact dermatitis is an inflammation resulting from direct contact with a substance to which the skin is sensitive. This could be an insect sting, poison ivy, cosmetics, soaps, or chemicals. The main symptom of contact dermatitis is urticaria. The treatment is a protective astringent lotion to prevent itching, dry up oozing, and guard against infections. For serious cases, an oral antihistamine may be given to counteract the allergic reaction and itching.

Eczema (Dermatitis). This is an inflammation with eruptions of pimplelike bumps, blisters, scales, or scabs. The lesions may be dry or "weepy" (having a watery discharge).

Eczema is a set of symptoms rather than a disease in itself. It is characterized by redness, swelling, itching, and a feeling of warmth to the touch. Eczema can be a reaction to a drug or a common substance. Creams, lotions, and ointments containing corticosteroids help suppress the inflammation of eczema. Oral antihistamines may be given instead, as eczema patients often develop sensitivity to the topical preparations.

◆ SYMPTOMS OF SKIN DISORDERS ◆ ◆ ◆

- **Pruritus** (itching)—caused by the release of histamine from the skin cells during allergic reactions.
- **Erythema** (reddening)—caused by an expansion of the capillaries close to the skin surface.
- **Edema** (swelling)—caused by a buildup of fluid in the spaces between cells due to inflammation.
- **Scaling**—an excess of a protein, keratin, in the epidermis. When a layer of dead cells builds up and becomes hard, the resulting condition is called **keratosis.**
- **Lesions**—patches, rashes, tumors, and sores that are flat or raised and appear in various colors, shapes, and sizes.
- **Ulcerations**—open lesions that are the result of tissue damage that starts below the skin and then erupts onto the skin surface.
- **Hives** or welts (urticaria)—raised, whitish patches that look like large mosquito bites and itch intensely. Hives can appear on parts of the body or cover the whole body. They are caused by a sensitivity to some substance in the environment or by various other factors such as fatigue and emotions.

Psoriasis. A chronic (long-term) skin condition, psoriasis is identified by its bright red, raised lesions covered with dry, silvery scales. The cause is unknown. It appears mainly on the knees, the elbows, the lower back, the scalp, the nails, the backs of the hands, the ears, the genitals, and the skin around the anus. Topical medications that are mildly irritating (keratolytics) are applied to the lesions. This mild irritation stimulates the healing of the underlying tissues. Psoriasis is also relieved by drugs that fight inflammation, such as corticosteroids.

Acne. Acne lesions develop in adolescence when growth hormones speed up the secretions of the oil (sebaceous) glands. The open pores of the skin become plugged with oil (sebum) and dead cells. This produces blackheads that can become inflamed. Treatment consists of cleansing with soap and water or an alcohol sponge. Topical preparations for acne include keratolytic drugs that produce peeling and open up the plugged pores. Tetracycline may be ordered by the physician to prevent infection or control the excess production of sebum.

Seborrheic Dermatitis. Seborrheic dermatitis is an inflammation of the scalp, face, or scrotum—areas that contain many sebaceous glands. Greasy scales are produced on lesions of the skin. Dry, white scales on the scalp are signs of a familiar noninflammatory variation of seborrhea called **dandruff.** Frequent washing and shampooing help to control seborrheic dermatitis or dandruff. Selenium sulfide keratolytics such as salicylic acid, zinc compounds (e.g., zinc pyrithione), and oral or topical corticosteroids are also used.

Burns. Burns can be mild or severe. They are caused by overexposure to sun, fire, steam, radiation, X rays, chemicals, or electricity. Mild burns (first-degree burns) merely redden the skin. More severe burns can blister the skin (second-degree burns). The most severe types of burns (third-degree burns) destroy underlying tissues. These burns have a charred or pearly white appearance. The treatment of serious burns is difficult and complex. A physician must order the proper treatment.

Mild astringents and cooling medications such as aluminum acetate are used for minor burns such as sunburn. Topical anti-infectives used for burns are mafenide *(Sulfamylon),* silver sulfadiazine, and gentamicin sulfate *(Garamycin).* These are applied as protective creams.

Patients who are sensitive to the sun may develop skin cancer after long periods of exposure. To prevent this, sunscreen products, such as oxybenzone cream *(Solbar)* are available. Para-aminobenzoic acid (PABA) is used for protection by individuals desiring a tan.

Decubitus Ulcers. Decubitus ulcers are bedsores caused by prolonged pressure between a body part and a hard or semihard surface. This condition occurs in patients who lie in bed for long periods of time without moving. The bedsores develop where the body is in contact with the bed (e.g., at the elbows, heels, and hips). The weight of the body presses down on these spots and shuts off blood circulation. Without oxygen and nutrients, the cells die and decay. The results are deep ulcerations.

Prevention is the best cure for bedsores. Once the tissues begin to break down, it becomes very difficult for the area to heal. Lotions may be rubbed into pressure spots to stimulate blood flow. Plastic coatings, substances that digest pus and clear wounds, and anti-inflammatory agents are sometimes administered topically around the sores.

Infections. Skin infections are caused by microbes invading the skin tissues. They may enter through a break in the skin. Or they may attack when the skin's natural protective chemistry is unbalanced. The signs of infection are the same as those of inflammation: reddening, swelling, warmth to the touch, and pain. In bacterial skin infections there is usually also pus, a thick, yellowish fluid made of dead white blood cells and debris. Impetigo and boils are examples of bacterial infections.

In fungus infections the skin is invaded by **fungi,** which are one-celled parasitic plants. Some common fungus infections are *tinea pedis* ("athlete's foot"), *tinea capitis* (ringworm of the scalp), and *tinea cruris* (ringworm of the groin, or "jock itch").

Fungal organisms can also develop in the mouth, around the anus, and in the vagina, causing itching and burning. Sometimes this happens after an antibiotic has been given orally to treat another disease. The antibiotic kills the helpful bacteria that usually destroy the fungus in these areas, causing superinfection.

Topical antiseptics and anti-infectives (antibiotics and antifungals) are designed to kill invading microbes on skin surfaces. Oral anti-infectives are also used.

Scabies and Pediculosis. Small insects called mites and lice cause these infestations. The mites of the disease scabies burrow under the skin. A month later the patient begins to develop symptoms such as watery blisters between the fingers. The infestation spreads very quickly. Special topical insecticides called **scabicides** are used to destroy the mites. There is no easy or fast treatment for scabies because the mites are very hard to eliminate. Bedding and clothing must be treated to help destroy the mites.

Pediculosis is caused by lice. These are insect parasites that lay eggs at the base of the hair of the head, in the pubic area, or in the seams of undergarments. Drugs called **pediculicides** are available to kill the lice. But all clothing, combs, and bedding must also be cleaned to help cure the condition. Patients must practice good hygiene if they want to avoid repeated infection.

TOPICAL MEDICATIONS

Major Categories

Each skin disorder has its own best treatment and drugs. But many of the drugs have things in common with each other. They belong to certain general categories or drug groups. If you learn what these categories are, you will understand how many drugs operate. For instance, suppose that you know that a particular drug is in the category "anti-infective." You then know that it works something like other anti-infectives you have studied in Chapter 6. Memorize the technical terms for these drug categories. This will help you especially when you are looking up drugs in drug reference books.

Oral drugs such as sedatives, antihistamines, and analgesics are sometimes ordered to make patients with skin diseases more comfortable. These oral drugs are described in other chapters. Most topical drugs for the skin fall into one or more of the following drug groups.

Keratolytics. Keratolytic drugs soften and destroy the outer layer of skin so that it is sloughed off (shed) (Figure 7-2). The name of this drug category comes from **keratin,** the protein found in the dead cells of the outer skin. Strong keratolytics are effective for removing warts and corns. Milder preparations are used to promote the shedding of scales and crusts in eczema, psoriasis, and seborrheic dermatitis. Very weak keratolytics irritate inflamed skin, which speeds up healing. Common keratolytics are salicylic acid, resorcinol, sulfur, and urea.

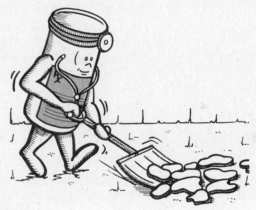

Figure 7-2   Keratolytics.

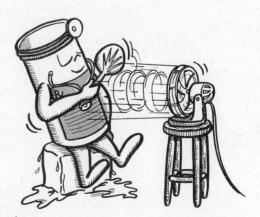

Figure 7-3   Protectives.

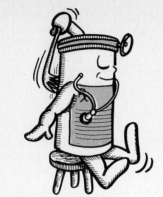

Figure 7-4 Antipruritics.

Protectives and Astringents. These drugs work by covering, cooling, drying, or soothing inflamed skin (Figure 7-3). Protectives do not penetrate the skin or soften it, but instead form a long-lasting film. This protects the skin from air, water, and clothing while the natural healing processes go on. Astringents shrink the blood vessels locally, dry up secretions from weepy lesions, and lessen the sensitivity of the skin.

Antipruritics. These drugs relieve itching caused by inflammation (Figure 7-4). Some of the drug forms themselves (e.g., emollients oils, creams, lotions) are soothing and thus help to relieve itching. **Corticosteroid** drugs (described later) relieve itching by suppressing the inflammation itself. **Antihistaminic drugs,** such as diphenhydramine *(Benadryl)* and hydroxyzine *(Atarax),* lessen the effects of **histamine,** the cause of the itching.

Anti-Inflammatory Drugs (Topical Corticosteroids). The corticosteroids have three actions that relieve symptoms of skin disorders:

- **Antipruritic**—relieves itching.
- **Anti-inflammatory**—suppresses the body's natural reactions to irritation.
- **Vasoconstrictive/venous insufficiency treatment**—tightens the blood vessels in the area of the inflammation. This reduces the swelling due to edema.

Most of the top-selling prescription drugs for the skin are corticosteroids. Examples are hydrocortisone, betamethasone *(Valisone, Celestone, Diprosone),* triamcinolone *(Aristocort, Kenalog),* fluocinonide *(Lidex),* fluocinolone acetate *(Synalar),* and flurandrenolide *(Cordran).* Vasoconstrictors or venous insufficiency treatment drugs are *Debrisan* beads or paste and *DuoDERM/Hydroactive* paste. The actions of corticosteroids are further described in Chapter 13.

Anti-Infectives (Antibacterials and Antifungals). These kill or inhibit microbes that cause skin infections. They also kill germs that enter the body through breaks in the skin surface and cause diseases. A few antibacterials are applied topically, but most are given systemically (see Chapter 6). Many common topical antibacterials are combinations of neomycin sulfate, polymyxin B, and bacitracin (e.g., *Neosporin, Neo-Polycin, Cortisporin).* Two soothing anti-infective preparations for burns are mafenide acetate *(Sulfamylon)* and silver sulfadiazine *(Silvadene).*

Antifungals (fungicides) are anti-infectives that treat specific fungus infections both by

- stopping the growth of fungus organisms and
- changing the condition of the skin cells so that fungi can no longer grow there.

Different antifungals are effective for different types of fungi. Fungus infections of the mouth, anus, and vagina are treated with such drugs as amphotericin B *(Fungizone),* nystatin *(Mycostatin),* and nystatin–triamcinolone–gramicidin *(Mycolog).* Preparations for ringworm and athlete's foot include clotrimazole *(Lotrimin),* tolnaftate *(Tinactin),* zinc undecylenate *(Desenex, Cruex),* and benzoic and salicylic acids. Griseofulvin *(Fulvicin P/G)* is given orally for severe cases that do not respond to topical medication.

Antiseptics. Antiseptics, such as alcohol, benzalkonium chloride *(Zephiran),* thimerosal *(Merthiolate),* mercurochrome, and povidone-iodine *(Betadine),* inhibit germs on skin surfaces. They are used topically, never given orally. Antiseptics prevent infections in cuts, scratches, and surgical wounds. (Disinfectants are very strong germ-killing drugs that are used only on nonliving objects such as surgical tools.)

Topical Anesthetics. For pain on the skin surfaces or mucous membranes, as in wounds, hemorrhoids, and sunburns, the physician may order a topical anesthetic. These relieve pain and itching by numbing the skin layers and mucous

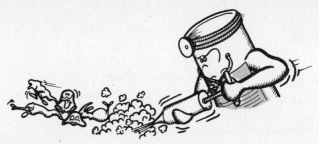

Figure 7-5 Parasiticides.

membranes. They are applied directly to the painful areas by means of sprays, creams, and suppositories. Examples are benzocaine *(Solarcaine)* and dibucaine *(Nupercainal)*.

Parasiticides. These are drugs that kill insect parasites that infest the skin (Figure 7-5). Scabicides kill the mites that cause scabies. Pediculicides kill the lice that cause pediculosis. A parasiticide that is effective against both scabies and lice is lindane *(Kwell)*.

The product information table at the end of this chapter lists a few representative drugs for treating skin disorders. The chart lists the drug category to which each drug belongs, its uses, actions hints for application, and side effects. As a giver of medications, you will be administering these drugs frequently. Be sure to consult your drug references and package inserts when you have questions or need additional information.

Table 7-1 lists some skin preparations available without a prescription. This list is provided for your information, as you are certain to handle these drugs regularly.

Transdermal Delivery System. Many prescription drugs that have for years been taken orally are now made in patch form to be absorbed into the bloodstream through the skin. People find the patch an easy and convenient way to take their medicine. For example, people with high blood pressure may use a clonidine patch *(Catapres-TTS)*. Other patches or transdermal delivery system drugs include nitroglycerin *(Nitro-Dur, Transderm-Nitro)* and estrogen. People

TABLE 7-1: Selected OTC Drugs for the Skin

CONDITION	PRODUCTS	ACTION
Acne	*Cuticura Medicated, Clearasil, Stri-Dex Medicated Pads*	Keratolytic
Dandruff	*Selsun Blue, Head and Shoulders, Sebisol*	Keratolytic/cytostatic
Diaper rash and prickly heat	*A & D Ointment, Desitin, Vaseline, Baby Magic, Johnson's Medicated Powder, zinc oxide*	Protective/antimicrobial
Dry skin	*Keri, Corn Huskers*	Emollient
Eczema and psoriasis	*Tegrin, Psorex, Zetar*	Keratolytic/antipruritic
Foot care	*Desenex, NP 27, Tinactin, Freezone*	Antifungal/keratolytic
Insect bites and stings	*Dermoplast, Nupercainal*	Anesthetic/antipruritic
Minor burns	*Medi-Quick, Solarcaine, Unguentine, Noxema*	Anesthetic/antimicrobial
Minor wounds	*Betadine, Zephiran Chloride, Baciguent, Neosporin, Neo-Polycin, Mycitracin*	Antiseptic/antibiotic
Poison ivy and poison oak	*Calamine, Caladryl, Ivy Dry Cream, Ziradryl*	Antipruritic/antihistaminic

who are trying to stop smoking cigarettes may be prescribed nicotine patches *(Nicoderm, Habitrol)*.

An important part of applying drug patches is marking the date and the time the patch was applied to the patient's skin. Also, when applying a new patch, remove the old patch first. More than one drug patch left on a patient can cause a possible overdose.

Absorption of Drugs into the Skin Layers

Drugs for the skin are prepared in the form of powders, lotions, gels, creams, ointments, pastes, and plasters. To refresh your memory about these forms of topical applications, review Chapter 3. The form that is chosen for a topically administered drug depends on the desired therapeutic effect.

The form affects the absorption of the drug into the deeper skin layers. Very few drugs used on the skin are supposed to be absorbed into the bloodstream unless they are delivered via the transdermal delivery system. Some, like the protectives and the antiseptics, are supposed to remain only on the skin surface. Others are designed to sink into the dermal and subcutaneous layers to provide anti-inflammatory or soothing actions. The type of drug, its form, and the nursing treatment that goes with it must be chosen very carefully by the physician to achieve the proper effect.

When absorption into the underlying skin layers is desired, the following measures increase absorption:

- *Apply wet dressings.* These bandages soften or macerate the skin. This permits the drug to pass through the epidermis, which is normally "waterproof."

- *Use a drug in an oil base.* The drug is absorbed easily through the pores of the sebaceous glands because the oil and the sebum blend together.

- *Rub the preparation into the skin.* This is done only when the skin is not covered with lesions that could be damaged by rubbing. Creams are rubbed in gently. Liniments are rubbed in vigorously. Hard rubbing also stimulates the skin, which draws blood to the area.

- *Keep medicine in contact with skin for a long time.* One way to achieve this is to cover the area with a dressing that prevents the drug from being rubbed off by sheets or clothing. Another way is to reapply the medication as soon as it seems to have worn off.

- *Apply an occlusive dressing if ordered by the physician.* An **occlusive bandage** does not permit evaporation of the drug. It holds the drug against the skin while at the same time holding in moisture so that the skin becomes **macerated** and readily absorbs the drug. An occlusive dressing holds in body heat, too, which increases absorption into the skin.

- *Use a stronger concentration of the drug.* When a preparation has more of the drug in it, there is more drug to be absorbed.

♦ **NOTE** ♦ ♦ ♦ ♦ ♦ ♦ ♦ ♦ ♦ ♦ ♦ ♦ ♦ ♦ ♦ ♦ ♦ ♦

Mucous membranes are treated very differently than skin when administering medications. These membranes make up the linings of body tubes and openings such as the mouth, the eyes, the rectum, and the vagina. Unlike the skin, the mucous membranes do not have a tough outer layer of dead cells to protect the underlying tissues. Instead, their surfaces are moist and easily penetrated. Therefore, drug absorption through the mucous membranes is very rapid. Topical preparations for the skin are formulated differently than those for mucous membranes. Never apply skin medications on mucous membranes, accidently or otherwise; this invites the risk of overmedicating the patient.

TABLE 7-2: Drug Categories for the Skin

Dermatologicals
Acne preparations
Analgesics
Antibacterials, antifungals, and
    combinations
Antibiotics
Anti-inflammatory agents
Astringents
Burn relief medications
Dandruff medications
Dermatitis relief medications
Drying agents
Keratolytics
Pediculicides
Pruritus medications

Psoriasis agents
Seborrhea treatments
Skin protectants
Steroids and combinations
Sunscreens
Wart removers
Wound cleansers
Wound dressings

Antiparasitics
Arthropods
    Lice
    Scabies

Absorption into the skin is most complete when several of these techniques are used at the same time—for example, a strong preparation held against the skin for a long period of time under an occlusive dressing. Absorption is also deeper in young children and elderly patients because these groups have thinner layers of skin.

Drugs applied to the skin are rarely supposed to be absorbed into the bloodstream. However, if the skin is cut, scratched, or scraped, or if there were many open sores, the drug may readily enter the bloodstream. This is usually undesirable and can be dangerous. Thus, to avoid poisoning the body with too high a dose of the drug, you will sometimes need to apply a preparation only at the base of a lesion or only around the infected area.

As you can see, the safe and effective absorption of each drug depends on many factors. For this reason, it is very important that you understand and follow instructions when applying each topical medication.

GENERAL INSTRUCTIONS FOR MEDICATING THE SKIN

Psychological Support

People who have skin conditions need your psychological support. Living with constant itching or pain is stressful. Patients may lose sleep because they cannot be comfortable. They may become depressed about their condition, especially if it lasts for a long time. This may have an effect on their appetite and intake of fluids.

Because of the psychological problems associated with skin diseases, doctors sometimes prescribe sedatives and tranquilizers. Patients with conditions like psoriasis, for which there is no permanent cure, may need counseling to help them live with the disease.

You can help these patients by accepting their feelings and responding to their needs with patience and understanding.

Patient Considerations

If the condition is painful, the doctor may have ordered an analgesic (pain-killing) drug. It is a good idea to plan to apply topical medications after a dose of analgesic so that you cause as little discomfort as possible.

Before giving the medication, explain to the patient what you are going to do. Inform him or her of any unusual sensations the drug may cause. For example, some gels produce warmth or a burning sensation on the skin.

Find a position that is comfortable for the patient and that lets you easily reach the skin area you need to work on. Protective pads should be placed under the affected area to keep the bed and the patient's clothing clean. (Some skin medications cause stains.) If possible, position the affected area so that the patient does not see it while you are applying the medication. Afterward, be sure to help the patient back into a normal position.

Wound Preparation

As lesions heal, the fluids that are produced dry out and form granules or crusts on the skin surface. These may be removed before applying medications, if ordered. This can be done by gently swabbing the crusts with sterile water. Or it can be done by soaking the area with hydrogen peroxide and then lifting the crusts away with forceps (surgical tweezers). The best way to clean the skin depends on the specific disease. In some cases you will also need to remove some of the dead skin with sterile forceps or scissors. This lets the medicine come in contact with live tissues so as to promote healing.

Apply medications only on the affected area. In the case of irritating substances, such as corn and wart removers, the healthy skin surrounding the lesions needs to be protected. A film of petroleum jelly provides good protection against absorption and irritation.

Some drugs must be diluted (mixed with water or some other liquid) before being applied. Follow instructions carefully to prepare the drug. Check with the pharmacy if you do not understand the directions. A drug that is improperly diluted could cause irritation or poisoning or be ineffective.

Applying the Medication

Apply the drugs as directed. In general, creams and liniments are rubbed in by hand. Lotions are patted on the skin with pieces of cotton. Ointments are applied with a wooden tongue blade or cotton swab (Figure 7-6). When infection or an open wound is present, you should use a sterile plastic glove. Apply the medication with a firm touch to avoid the sensation of itching.

When opening the container, place the cap upside down on the medicine tray or cart. Use a sterile tongue blade or cotton swab to dip out a quantity of medication from its container. Do not dip in and out with the same applicator you are using on the patient! Then apply the medication according to instructions (the physician's or those in the package insert). See Practice Procedure 7-1.

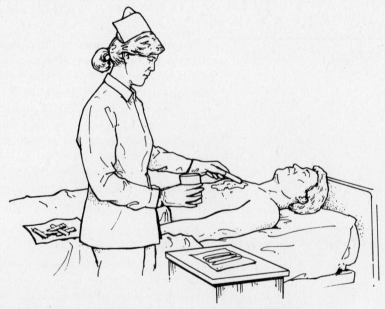

Figure 7-6 Applying medication with a wooden tongue blade.

When medicating large areas, work on one section at a time and drape the remaining parts of the body with sheets. Work systematically, using a pattern to help you cover the entire area. For example, you might use a circular motion or a back-and-forth motion.

A few skin drugs are administered by means of a medicated bath (e.g., a coal tar for a psoriasis patient), a special soap or shampoo (e.g., acne soaps, pediculicides), or an injection directly into a lesion. For specific instructions on the nursing care that goes with these drugs, refer to a manual of nursing procedures.

The instruction "Apply as needed" is given only for drugs that carry no danger of overdose. Reapply the medication whenever the symptoms flare up, or when the thin film of drug has worn off or has been absorbed into the skin. A registered nurse or physician is frequently responsible for deciding when to reapply the medication. Others may do so if they have the permission of the physician or nurse.

Bandages and Dressings

Bandages and other coverings should be used only when ordered by the physician. This is because they hold in body heat and increase absorption. Some lesions must be covered to protect them from clothing and scratching. Others must be covered to keep the medication in constant contact with the affected skin. However, a bandage can be irritating rather than helpful. Many lesions heal better when left exposed to air.

Infected lesions that are actively producing pus are usually bandaged to soak up the fluids. The bandages must be changed frequently.

Care must be taken when removing bandages from a wound so as to avoid pulling away the scab. A dressing that is sticking to a lesion may be softened by moistening it with sterile water. To avoid removing and reapplying tape each time a dressing is changed, you may use butterfly tape strips.

Follow-Up

Charting Observations. Each time you prepare to apply a topical medication, make a note of the appearance of the skin. Has there been a change for better or for worse since you last saw it? If there is no change, then perhaps the medication is not working. Are there any signs of irritation? Be sure to chart your observations, since these will help in evaluating the patient's progress and pinpointing problems.

Side Effects. Be on the lookout for any signs of irritation that do not seem to come from the disease itself. Many persons are sensitive to certain drugs. They may develop rashes, dryness, redness, tiny purplish-red spots, and ruptures of surface blood vessels (**petechiae, ecchymosis**), sensitivity to light (**photodermatitis**), and/or itching in the area where you applied the medication. These signs should be charted and reported to the nurse in charge. The strength of the drug may be changed or another drug or treatment may be ordered.

Patient Education. Instruct your patients in how to apply skin medications properly. If there is a long-lasting condition, they will be responsible for their own skin care. The PDR is a good place to look for information that will be useful to the patient.

CATEGORY, NAME[a], AND ROUTE	USES AND DISEASES	ACTIONS	USUAL DOSE[b] AND SPECIAL INSTRUCTIONS	SIDE EFFECTS AND ADVERSE REACTIONS
Keratolytics				
Salicylic acid Topical	Seborrheic dermatitis, psoriasis, warts, corns, calluses	Swells and softens excess keratin for easy removal or shedding	Dosage depends on form and strength of preparation. Soaking skin before use assists drug action. Apply dressing as ordered. Do not put drug in contact with eyes, mucous membranes, or normal skin	Irritation, burning
Carbol-fuchsin (Castellani's Paint) Topical	Antifungal agent for athlete's foot and ringworm infections	Kills fungus on contact	Apply to affected area once or twice a day	Irritation of affected area
Astringents				
Calamine and diphenhydramine (Caladryl) Lotion	Itching from poison ivy or poison oak, insect bites, or other skin irritations; mild sunburn	Relief of itching; soothes mild sunburns; drying action	Apply topically 3 or 4 times daily. Clean and dry area before applying	Burning or itching; consult doctor
Antipruritics				
Trimeprazine tartrate (Temaril) Oral	Urticaria, atopic and contact dermatitis, pityriasis rosea, and drug rash	Relief of itching; is an antihistamine and antipruritic; has a drying effect and a sedative effect	2.5 mg 4 times daily; 1 spansule q12h	*Short-term therapy:* drowsiness, hypotension, bradycardia, faintness, and very rarely, anorexia, nausea, and vomiting, dry mouth *Long-term therapy:* skin pigmentation, extrapyramidal reactions (dyskinesia)

◆◆

CATEGORY, NAME[a], AND ROUTE	USES AND DISEASES	ACTIONS	USUAL DOSE[b] AND SPECIAL INSTRUCTIONS	SIDE EFFECTS AND ADVERSE REACTIONS
Anti-Inflammatory Drugs (Topical Corticosteroids)				
Betamethasone valerate *(Valisone)* Topical	Contact dermatitis, dermatoses, psoriasis	Suppresses inflammation, relieves itching and swelling	Dosage depends on form and strength of preparation. Apply ointment, lotion, or cream sparingly and massage gently into affected area. Do not apply in or near eyes. Also available as aerosol; do not inhale spray. Check skin regularly for signs of irritation. Use occlusive dressing as ordered	Irritation, burning, itching, blistering, peeling
Triamcinolone *(Aristocort)* Topical	Contact dermatitis, oral lesions	Suppresses inflammation, relieves itching and swelling	Dose varies depending on condition	Irritation, burning, itching, blistering, peeling
Hydrocortisone OTC: *Hytone* 0.5% ointment *Delacort* 0.5% lotion *Bactine* 0.5% cream *Aeroseb HC* 0.5% spray *Cortef Rectal Itch* 0.5% ointment	OTC: Temporary relief of many minor skin, genital, and anal itching and rashes; anorectal products used for severe inflammation and swelling have other ingredients such as belladonna and benzocaine	Anti-inflammatory, antipruritic, and vasoconstrictive actions	Use sparingly and rub in lightly. Cover *only as directed* with occlusive dressing Protect patient's face when spraying with aerosols and avoid inhalation when using this form of medication	Burning and itching sensations, irritation, dryness and skin maceration, especially if used with occlusive dressings. Systemic effects may occur if used excessively or for a prolonged time
Prescription: *Dermacort* 1.0% lotion *Synacort* 2.5% cream *Sensacort* 0.5% spray *Nutracort* 1.0% gel *Cort-Dome* 15 mg suppositories *Proctofoam* 1.0% aerosol foam	Prescription: Relief of inflammatory and pruritic manifestations of corticosteroid-responsive dermatosis			

◆◆

CATEGORY, NAME[a], AND ROUTE	USES AND DISEASES	ACTIONS	USUAL DOSE[b] AND SPECIAL INSTRUCTIONS	SIDE EFFECTS AND ADVERSE REACTIONS
Anti-Infectives, Antibacterials, Antifungals				
Mafenide acetate *(Sulfamylon)* Topical	Burns	Antibacterial, soothes and protects	Cleanse area of debris before application. Apply with sterile tongue blade or gloved hand to a thickness of 1/16th inch. Keep area covered with medication at all times. Apply dressing as ordered	Pain, burning, stinging, allergic reactions, fungal superinfection
Clotrimazole *(Lotrimin)* Topical	Fungus infections, ringworm, athlete's foot	Antifungal, relieves itching	Gently massage into affected area twice a day, morning and night	Redness, urticaria, irritation
Griseofulvin *(Fulvicin)* Oral	Severe fungus or infections of hair, skin, and nails	Antifungal	500–1000 mg/day (microsize) PO in single or divided doses. Caution patient to avoid sunlight. Give after meal with high fat content to increase absorption	Headache, photosensitivity
Nystatin *(Mycostatin)* Topical	Cutaneous or mucocutaneous mycotic infections caused by *Candida* (Monilia) *albicans*	Fungistatic and fungicidal against a wide variety of yeast fungi	Apply cream and ointment liberally to affected area twice daily or as indicated until healing is complete; powder should be applied to the lesion 2 or 3 times daily until lesion is healed	Irritation possible but well tolerated even by infants
1% silver sulfadiazine *(Silvadene)* Topical cream	Adjunct for prevention and treatment of wound sepsis in second- and third-degree burns	Antibacterial and antimicrobial	Cleanse and debride; cover with drug at all times. Reapply 1 or 2 times daily using sterile technique to a thickness of 1/16th inch	Itching, burning, or rash; adverse reactions attributed to sulfonamides

◆◆

Vasoconstrictors/Venous Insufficiency Treatments

Debrisan Topical paste and beads	Adjunct treatment of wet ulcer (e.g., decubitus ulcers)	Reduces swelling and edema; increases venous flow	Dosage depends on strength of beads or paste. Packets are 25–60 g each; paste available in 10-g foil packets	Pain, transitory bleeding, blistering, erythema
DuoDERM hydroactive Granules/beads, paste	Dermal exudating ulcers; dermal ulcers	Local management of ulcer by forming a gellike substance of the moisture in ulcers or wounds	Sterile 30-g tube; avoid use when muscle, bone, or tendon is involved; do not use on pressure sores, ulcers from tuberculosis or deep fungal infections	Infection; odor or change in color due to infection; fever, cellulitis

Antiseptics

Povidone-iodine *(Betadine)* Topical	Surface infections, burns, minor wounds, vaginitis	Kills germs	Apply as ordered; avoid contact with eyes	Irritation, redness, swelling

Anesthetics

Benzocaine *(Solarcaine)* Topical	Pruritus, minor burns; oral, nasal, and gingival mucous membranes	Inhibits conduction of nerve impulses from sensory nerves	Give smallest effective dose according to age	Sensitization

a   Product names given in parentheses are examples only. Check current drug references for a complete listing of available products.

b   Average adult doses are given. However, dosages are determined by a physician and vary with the purpose of the therapy and the particular patient. The doses presented in this text are for general information only.

◆◆

● ● ● PRACTICE PROCEDURE 7-1 ● ● ●

Applying Topical Medication to the Skin

Equipment

- Sterile gloves
- Sterile scissors, forceps
- Sterile dressings and coverings
- Sterile applicators: tongue blades, gauze, cotton balls, or swabs
- Medication (lotion, ointment, cream, liniment, or aerosol spray)
- Bag or newspapers for disposal
- Medication record, Kardex, medicine card, or the form used by your agency

Procedure

1. Assemble equipment, medications, and patients' records.

2. Read the Kardex, medication record, or medicine card. Check this information against the medication label. Be sure you have the RIGHT DRUG and the RIGHT DOSE for the RIGHT PATIENT at the RIGHT TIME by the RIGHT ROUTE.

3. Read the instructions on application in the package insert.

4. Identify the patient and explain the procedure. Check the patient's wrist ID or follow agency policy for identifying patients.

5. Administer a systemic analgesic (if ordered) to relieve pain caused by applying topical medication. Wait for 10–20 minutes.

6. Position the patient and the affected area comfortably. Protect clothing and bed linen with pads, if necessary.

7. Wash your hands.

8. Open the gloves, dressings, applicators, and medication needed. The lid of the medication container should be placed upside down on the table or tray to avoid contaminating the medication. Then put on sterile gloves to prevent wound contamination.

9. Remove old, soiled dressings. Discard them in a newspaper or disposal bag. Be careful not to pull the scab off a newly healed area. If the dressing sticks to the wound, apply sterile water. Let it soak for 5–10 minutes.

10. Cleanse and remove dead tissue or crusts from lesions if ordered. Use a cleansing liquid ordered by the physician. Remove dead tissue with sterile scissors or forceps. Remove crusts with cotton swabs or forceps.

11. Reread the label to make sure that you have the right drug.

12. Take medication from its container using a sterile applicator (tongue blade or swab). Try to dip out the entire amount you will need for one application.

13. Apply the medication using the correct procedure for the medication form.
    - Creams: rub in gently.
    - Lotions: pat or dab on skin.
    - Liniments: rub in vigorously.
    - Ointments: apply with a wooden blade or cotton swab.
    - Aerosol sprays: hold the can upright and spray the area from a distance of 3–6 inches; spray a second and a third time.
    - Foam medication: hold the can inverted next to the skin and spray.
    - Beads: mix with a suitable substance (e.g., glycerin) and apply directly to the wound with a sterile wooden spatula.
    - Paste: swab piercing (on cap) with alcohol and remove it; puncture the tube by inverting the cap back into the tube; squeeze paste onto the wound.

14. Apply a thin or thick amount (one-fourth of the thickness for paste or beads) as ordered by the physician or as stated on the package directions. Be systematic in covering the affected area.

15. Cover the area with wet or dry dressings, if ordered. (See the doctor's orders, package insert, or procedure manual for instructions.) Secure dressings with adhesive tape or butterfly tape strips.

16. Instruct the patient in further care of the skin. See package directions or the doctor's orders. Remove your gloves.

17. Make the patient comfortable before leaving. Fluff pillows, return the patient to a normal position, secure call button, and so forth.

18. Remove, clean, and/or discard equipment and supplies. Put away medications, rereading the labels as you do so. Dispose of used supplies in the appropriate area. Wash your hands.

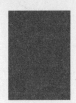

19. Record the application of medication. Note:
    - Condition of the skin or skin lesions (on nurses' notes).
    - Reactions of the patient (on nurses' notes).
    - Date, time, medication, and dosage (on medication record).

Demonstrate this procedure for your instructor or the nurse in charge.

CHAPTER 7 REVIEW

Using Medical Terminology

Match these skin structures to the jobs they do.

_____ 1. Ceruminous gland   a. secretes ear wax

_____ 2. Epidermis   b. grows hair

_____ 3. Hair follicle   c. secretes oil

_____ 4. Mammary gland   d. secretes sweat

_____ 5. Sebaceous gland   e. feels pressure or pain

_____ 6. Sense receptor   f. secretes milk

_____ 7. Subcutaneous   g. insulates and stores energy

_____ 8. Sudoriferous gland   h. acts as a waterproof covering

Define these medical terms.

9. Pruritus _____

10. Erythema _____

11. Edema _____

12. Keratin _____

13. Parasite _____

14. Lesion _____

15. Acne _____

16. Antiseptic _____

17. Dermis _____

18. Integument _____

19. Sebum _____

20. Ulceration _____

Acquiring Knowledge of Medications

Describe the purpose of the following types of drugs.

21. Antipruritics _____

22. Antiseptics _____

23. Topical corticosteroids _____

24. Topical anesthetics _____

25. Keratolytics _____

26. Parasiticides _____

27. Protectives _____

28. Astringents _____

29. Vasoconstrictors _____

30. Antibacterials _____

Place a check (✓) by the number next to each item known to increase the absorption of a drug into the layers of the skin.

_____ 31. Strong drug mixture   _____ 37. occlusive dressing

_____ 32. Dry dressing   _____ 38. very young or very old patient

_____ 33. Oil-based drug   _____ 39. patting drug on skin

_____ 34. Unbroken skin   _____ 40. rubbing drug into skin

_____ 35. Broken skin   _____ 41. giving an oral antihistamine

_____ 36. Wet dressing   _____ 42. reapplying drug when worn off

Match drug names to drug categories.

_____ 43. Salicylic acid, resorcinol   a. topical corticosteriods

_____ 44. *Aristocort, Valisone, Cordran*   b. parasiticide

_____ 45. *Tinactin, Mycostatin, Lotrimin*   c. topical anesthetics

_____ 46. *Kwell*   d. oral antipruritics

_____ 47. *Neosporin, Sulfamylon*   e. topical antibacterials

_____ 48. Zinc oxide, calamine   f. topical antifungals

_____ 49. *Temaril, Atarax*   g. antiseptics

_____ 50. Griseofulvin   h. keratolytics

_____ 51. *Betadine,* alcohol, *Merthiolate*   i. protectives and astringents

_____ 52. Benzocaine   j. oral antifungal

_____ 53. *Zithromax,* clarithromycin   k. vasoconstrictors

_____ 54. *Debrisan, Duo/DERM*   l. oral antibacterial

Place a + in the blank if the statement is true. Place a O in the blank if the statement is false.

_____ 55. For painful skin conditions, it is good to apply topical medications before giving a dose of pain reliever.

_____ 56. Patients with skin diseases need psychological support.

_____ 57. Try to position the patient so that he or she has a good view of the area you are medicating.

_____ 58. Do not explain medication procedures to patients unless they ask you to do so.

_____ 59. Remove crusts from lesions by rubbing them firmly with a cotton swab.

_____ 60. When using strong keratolytics on warts and corns, the surrounding healthy skin may be protected with petroleum jelly.

_____ 61. Creams and liniments should be rubbed in by hand.

_____ 62. If there is any ointment left on a wooden blade after application, you may scrape it off into the medication container.

_____ 63. When removing the cap of a medication jar or bottle, the cap should be placed upside down on the tray or cart.

_____ 64. Do not use a dressing unless ordered by the physician.

_____ 65. A sticky bandage should be softened with sterile water to avoid removing the scab.

Applying Knowledge on the Job

Select the skin disorder that best matches each description.

Decubitus   Pediculosis   Seborrheic dermatitis
Eczema (dermatitis)   Psoriasis   Tinea capitis

66. Mr. Yee has applied *Kwell* cream on his body to combat scabies. After a few hours his skin becomes dry and scaly. It is read, swollen, itchy, and warm to the touch.

_____

_____

67. Miss Barnett has suffered from dry scales on the backs of her hands for many years. The symptoms are kept under control with *Celestone*.

_____

_____

68. Fred Entler is annoyed to find dry, white, greasy scales on his scalp.

_____

_____

69. Fran Graham is bedridden with a muscle disease. A sore is developing where her tailbone touches the sheets.

_____

_____

70. Mr. Chopra's doctor says that this patient has ringworm of the scalp and orders griseofulvin to treat it.

_____

_____

71. While washing her children's hair, Mrs. Johnson discovers tiny eggs laid in their scalps at the base of the hairs.

_____

_____

Answer the questions below in the spaces provided.

72. Is it all right to use a skin medication on mucous membranes? Explain your answer.

_____

_____

_____

_____

_____

73. Before applying a topical medication, you are expected to examine the skin very carefully. What signs would you chart on the nurses' notes?

_____

_____

_____

_____

Using Resources on the Job

Obtain a current copy of the PDR from your school, nursing unit, or clinic. Use it to answer the following questions in a notebook or on file cards.

74. In Section 4 of the PDR, Generic and Chemical Name Index, find another product name for each of the categories of drugs listed on the chart Representative Drugs for the Skin on pages 166–169 of this text.

75. In Section 3 of the PDR, Product Category Index, find *Psoriasis Agents* (under Dermatologicals). List all the agents found there.

76. Section 3 lists page numbers for some agents shown in Section 5, Product Identification. List three drugs with Section 5 page numbers. Turn to the page numbers given and locate the pictures of three drugs used for psoriasis.

77. For the same three drugs you saw pictured, name the manufacturer. Use Section 1 of the PDR, Manufacturers' Index, to find the address of each manufacturer.

78. In Section 2 of the PDR, Product Name Index, identify the pages that provide information about these three drugs. Read about the drugs in Section 6, Product Information.

79. In Section 6, locate the information about each of the three drugs that refers to children and the elderly.

80. Use Section 7 of the PDR, Diagnostic Product Information, to find one of the manufacturers you identified in Question 77. List the diagnostic drugs produced by this manufacturer.

81. Summarize your findings in writing.

_____

_____

_____

_____

_____

_____

_____

_____

_____

_____

> If you have difficulty finding a drug in the PDR, turn to the back and look under *Discontinued Products* to see if it has been discontinued.

Using Medical Terminology

1. a 2. h 3. b
4. f 5. c 6. e
7. g 8. d
9. Itching
10. Redness
11. Swelling
12. Protein contained in cells of the epidermis, nails, hair, and horny tissue
13. Organism that lives on or in another organism
14. Cut, scrape, sore, or any change in the structure of a body part
15. Skin condition caused by pores being plugged with sebum
16. An agent that inhibits germs
17. Middle layer of skin
18. The skin
19. Oil in the skin
20. Open sore

Acquiring Knowledge of Medications

21. To relieve itching
22. To inhibit germs on surfaces
23. To suppress inflammation, relieve itching, and reduce swelling
24. To relieve pain on skin surfaces or mucous membranes
25. To soften hardened skin and promote peeling and shedding
26. To kill parasites such as mites and lice
27. To form a film over the skin
28. To shrink blood vessels
29. To tighten blood vessels, thus reducing swelling

30. To kill or inhibit microbe growth on skin
31. ✓ 32. — 33. ✓
34. — 35. ✓ 36. ✓
37. ✓ 38. ✓ 39. —
40. ✓ 41. — 42. ✓
43. h 44. a 45. f
46. b 47. e 48. i
49. d 50. j 51. g
52. c 53. l 54. k
55. 0 56. + 57. 0
58. 0 59. 0 60. +
61. + 62. 0 63. +
64. + 65. +

Applying Knowledge on the Job

66. Eczema (dermatitis)
67. Psoriasis
68. Seborrheic dermatitis
69. Decubitus
70. Tinea capitis
71. Pediculosis
72. Skin medications should not be used on mucous membranes because absorption is much quicker through mucous membranes than through skin.
73. Chart any changes in the condition of the skin since you last applied medication. Note dryness, rashes, redness, ecchymosis, petechiae, or any other sign of irritation that is not a symptom of the disease itself. Also, make a note if there seems to be *no* change for the better after several applications of the drug.

Using Resources on the Job

74–80. Answers will vary depending on the edition of the PDR used.

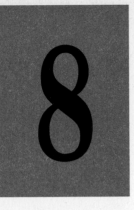

C
H
A
P
T
E
R

8

Drugs for the Cardiovascular System

◆◆ In this chapter you will learn about the organs and functions of the cardiovascular system and what goes wrong with them during common cardiovascular disorders. You will study the types of drugs used to treat each disorder and learn to classify common generic and product name drugs according to their drug categories. You will also practice step-by-step procedures for administering and sublingual medications.

COMPETENCIES

After studying this chapter, you should be able to

- name the parts of the cardiovascular system and state their functions.

- recognize the names of instruments used to measure blood pressure and to record the heartbeat.

- state the average blood pressure and pulse rate.

- list the main components of blood.

- state the functions of the lymphatic system.

- give the proper medical terms for common symptoms of cardiovascular disorders.

- recognize descriptions of the major disorders for which cardiovascular drugs are given.

- describe the actions and give examples of the following drug groups: vasoconstrictors, vasodilators, antihypertensives, heart stimulants/cardiac glycerides, arrhythmic medications (antiarrhythmics), anticoagulants, coagulants, hematinics, and thrombolytics.

- state the difference between a maintenance dose and an initial dose.

- follow the proper procedure for administering oral and sublingual medications to patients with cardiovascular disorders.

- state the special nursing procedures for administering vasoconstrictors, vasodilators, antihypertensives, digitalis, antiarrhythmics, anticoagulants, coagulants, and hematinics.